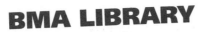
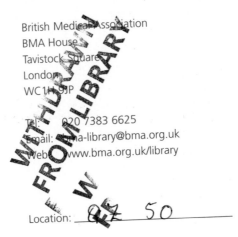

Lecture Notes
Medical Genetics

John R. Bradley
Department of Medicine
Cambridge University Hospitals NHS Foundation Trust
Cambridge, UK

David R. Johnson
Clinical Immunology Branch
National Institute of Allergy and Infections Diseases
National Institutes of Health, Bethesda, MD, USA

Barbara R. Pober
Department of Pediatrics
MassGeneral Hospital for Children
Department of Surgery
Children's Hospital
Boston, MA, USA

Third Edition

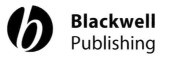
Blackwell
Publishing

© 2006 John R. Bradley, David R. Johnson, Barbara Pober
Published by Blackwell Publishing Ltd

Blackwell Publishing, Inc., 350 Main Street, Malden, Massachusetts 02148-5020, USA
Blackwell Publishing Ltd, 9600 Garsington Road, Oxford OX4 2DQ, UK
Blackwell Publishing Asia Pty Ltd, 550 Swanston Street, Carlton, Victoria 3053, Australia

First published 1995
Second edition 2001
Reprinted 2003
Third edition 2006

Library of Congress Cataloging-in-Publication Data

Data available

ISBN-13: 978-1-4051-3003-5
ISBN-10: 1-4051-3003-2

A catalogue record for this title is available from the British Library

Set in 8/12pts Stone Serif by NewGen Imaging Systems (P) Ltd, Chennai, India
Printed and bound by COS Printers Pte Ltd, Singapore

Commissioning Editor: Martin Sugden
Editorial Assistant: Caroline Boyd
Development Editor: Mirjana Misina
Production Controller: Kate Charman

For further information on Blackwell Publishing, visit our website:
http://www.blackwellpublishing.com

The publisher's policy is to use permanent paper from mills that operate a sustainable forestry policy, and which
has been manufactured from pulp processed using acid-free and elementary chlorine-free practices. Furthermore,
the publisher ensures that the text paper and cover board used have met acceptable environmental accreditation
standards.

Contents

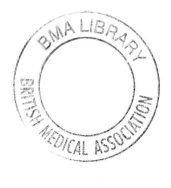

Preface

The first edition of Lecture Notes of Molecular Medicine was written at a time when the introduction of novel technologies to manipulate molecules led to a dramatic increase in our understanding of the molecular basis of disease. Hopes were raised that cures for many diseases would soon follow, with gene therapy leading the way. In practice the impact has been more subtle, but as important. Our understanding of the influence of genetic variation on disease processes has improved the prevention, detection and management of many conditions, and will inform the use of existing treatments and the development of new therapies. These advances are reflected in the new title and substance of the third edition of Lecture Notes on Medical Genetics.

List of Abbreviations

A	adenine
ACE	angiotensin converting enzyme
ACTH	adrenocorticotropic hormone
AD	Alzheimer disease
ADA	adenosine deaminase
AFB1	aflatoxin B1
AFP	alphafetoprotein
AIP	acute intermittent porphyria
ALA	aminolaevulinic acid
APC	adenomatosis polyposis coli
APP	amyloid precursor protein
ARMS	amplification refractory mutation system
AS	Angelman syndrome
ATP	adenosine triphosphate
BACs	bacterial artificial chromosomes
BLAST	basic local alignment search tool
BMT	bone marrow transplantation
bp	base pairs
BrdU	bromodeoxyuridine
C	cytosine
CAH	congenital adrenal hyperplasia
cDNA	complementary DNA
CFTR	cystic fibrosis transmembrane conductance regulator
CGH	comparative genomic hybridization
CK	creatine phosphokinase
cM	centimorgan
CML	chronic myeloid leukaemia
CMT	Charcot–Marie–Tooth
COMT	catechol-O-methyl transferase
CsCl	Caesium chloride
CVS	chorionic villus sampling
dADO	deoxyadenosine
dATP	deoxyadenosine triphosphate
ddNTPs	dideoxynucleotides
DHFR	dihydrofolate reductase
DMD	Duchenne muscular dystrophy
DMPK	myotonia-dystrophica protein kinase
DNA	deoxyribonucleic acid
dNTPs	deoxynucleotide triphosphates
DOP-PCR	degenerate oligonucleotide primed PCR
DRPLA	Dentatorubropallidoluysian atrophy
dsRNA	double-stranded RNA
EGFR	epidermal growth factor receptor
eIFs	elongation factors
ELSI	ethical, legal and social implications
EMG	electromyography
EMS	ethane methyl sulphonate
ENU	ethylnitrosourea
ERT	enzyme replacement therapy
ES	embryonic stem
EST	expressed sequence tag
EtBr	ethidium bromide
FAP	familial adenomatous polyposis
FISH	fluorescent in situ hybridization
FMF	familial Mediterranean fever
FRET	fluorescence resonance energy transfer
G	guanine
HATs	histone acetyl transferases
hCG	human chorionic gonadotrophin
HCM	hypertrophic cardiomyopathy
HDACs	histone deacetylases
HERVs	human endogenous retroviruses
HHT	hereditary haemorrhagic telangiectasia
HLA	human leucocyte antigen
HMSN	hereditary motor and sensory neuropathies
HNPCC	hereditary nonpolyposis colorectal cancer
HNPP	hereditary neuropathy with liability to pressure palsies
hnRNA	heterogeneous nuclear RNA
HSV-1	herpes simplex virus type-1
IDDM	insulin-dependent diabetes mellitus
IHF	integration host factor
IMGT	immunogenetics
Int	bacteriophage-encoded integrase

List of Abbreviations

IVS	intervening sequences
LCR	locus control region
LCV	large-scale copy-number variants
LD	linkage disequilibrium
LDL	low density lipoprotein
LINEs	long interspersed nuclear elements
LOD	logarithm of the odds
LTR	long terminal repeat
Mbp	millions of base pairs
MDA	multiple displacement amplification
MHC	major histocompatibility complex
miRNA	micro RNA
MMR	mismatch repair
MODY	maturity-onset diabetes of the young
MPS II	mucopolysaccharidoses type II
mRNA	messenger RNA
MSI	microsatellite instability
NF 1	neurofibromatosis type 1
NG	nitrosoguanidine
NIDDM	non-insulin-dependent diabetes mellitus
NIH	National Institutes of Health
OI	osteogenesis imperfecta
OMIM	online Mendelian inheritance in man
ORFs	open reading frames
PCR	polymerase chain reaction
PEG	polyethylene glycol
PFGE	pulsed field gel electrophoresis
PKU	phenylketonuria
pol	polymerase
PP	pyrophosphate
PT	prothrombin time
PTT	partial-thromboplastin time
PWS	Prader-Willi Syndrome
rAAV	recombinant adeno-associated viral vectors
RAC	Recombinant DNA Advisory Committee
RFLP	restriction fragment length polymorphism
RH	radiation hybrids
rhDNase	recombinant human deoxyribonuclease
RISC	RNA-induced silencing complex
R-M	restriction–modification
RNA	ribonucleic acid
RNAi	RNA interference
RNases	ribonucleases
RP	retinitis pigmentosa
rRNA	ribosomal RNA
S	Svedberg units
SAGE	serial analysis of gene expression
SCA12	Spinocerebellar Ataxia Type 12
SCID	severe combined immune deficiency
SDS	sodium dodecyl sulphate
SHOX	short structure homeobox
SINEs	short interspersed nuclear elements
siRNA	small interfering RNA
SLE	systemic lupus erythematosus
SMA	spinal muscular atrophy
SMN	survival motor neurone
SNPs	single nucleotide polymorphisms
SNRPN	small nuclear ribonucleoprotein N
STS	sequence-tagged site
SV40	simian virus 40
T	thymine
TdT	terminal deoxytransferase
TGF-β	transforming growth factor-β
TNT	trinucleotide
tRNA	transfer RNA
u	uracil
UFD1L	ubiquitin fusion degradation 1-like protein
UTR	untranslated region
UV	ultraviolet
VCF	velocardiofacial
VEGF	vascular endothelial growth factor
VNTR	variable numbers of tandem repeats
WASp	Wiskott–Aldrich syndrome protein
WGA	whole genome amplification
WHO	World Health Organization
Xis	excisionase
XIST	X-inactivation-specific transcript
XLD	X-linked dominant
YACs	yeast artificial chromosomes

Chapter 1

Basic principles

Viruses and bacteria have ensured their survival over millions of years by using a variety of techniques to make, break and join deoxynucleic acid (DNA) and ribonucleic acid (RNA). In recent years, molecular biologists have adapted and exploited these naturally occurring processes, leading to remarkable breakthroughs in understanding the molecular basis of human disease. Methods for manipulating the nucleic acids DNA and RNA are extensive, and protein methodology is developing rapidly. This chapter provides an overview of the molecules involved, with an emphasis on understanding some of the fundamental principles that underlie the rapidly evolving techniques used to study disease. A better grasp of the fundamental technology will help in appreciating the possibilities and identifying the limits of translating new discoveries in molecular medicine into diagnostic tests and therapies for patients.

Organisms are made of cells

Living organisms are composed of cells. Some organisms, including bacteria, algae and yeasts, exist as single cells, whereas plants and animals consist of collections of cells. New cells, required for growth of an existing organism or the formation of new organisms, arise by division of existing cells.

Cell functions depend on proteins

All cellular functions depend on proteins, which consist of chains of amino acids. Only 20 different amino acids are commonly found in the proteins of all organisms. The links in a chain of amino acids are termed peptide bonds and the chains themselves are called polypeptides. Proteins contain one or more polypeptides, and the structure and function of each protein depends on the sequence of amino acids making up the polypeptide chains.

Proteins have many diverse functions. They maintain cell structure and provide motility, act as intra- and extracellular messengers, and bind and transport molecules, including oxygen, lipids and other proteins. Many proteins are enzymes which catalyse (accelerate) chemical reactions. Almost all chemical reactions, including those involved in the synthesis of fats and carbohydrates, are catalysed by enzymes.

Some proteins, for example, the enzymes involved in glucose metabolism, are present in most cells. In contrast, cells in multicellular organisms may become specialized and produce certain proteins that provide them with highly specific functions. Cells that produce particular proteins are often grouped together to form complex tissues or organs. For example, muscle cells produce proteins, including tropomyosin and myosin, which are involved in the formation of muscle filaments, islet cells of the pancreas synthesize the polypeptide hormone insulin, and liver cells contain enzymes found exclusively in the liver, such as those required for the conjugation of bilirubin into water-soluble forms.

DNA contains the information needed to encode proteins

Cells therefore need:

• the information to produce proteins in a regulated fashion;
• the ability to convey this information to daughter cells during cell division.

The key to these requirements is provided by the *DNA double helix*, which contains two strands of DNA held together by weak chemical interactions.

Basic DNA Structure

Each strand of DNA has a backbone of sugars and phosphates, with a nitrogen-containing base attached to each sugar. Four different bases are found in DNA. Cytosine (C) and thymine (T) are pyrimidines which contain one nitrogenous ring, whereas adenine (A) and guanine (G) are purines which contain two. The bases from each strand are linked together to form the 'rungs' inside the helix in such a way that A can only pair with T, and C can only pair with G (Figure 1.1). In RNA the sugar is ribose, uracil replaces T and the resulting nucleic acid is single stranded.

The strands complement each other – the sequences of bases on one strand can be determined from the sequence of the other strand. During cell division each strand independently forms a new complementary strand and the DNA helix is able to direct its own duplication.

The sequence of bases in a DNA molecule carries the information that specifies the order of amino acids along a polypeptide chain. Each of the 20 amino acids is encoded by coding units, or codons, which consist of three consecutive bases. Reading this code and translating it into protein requires RNA.

A segment of DNA that carries the information needed to encode a specific polypeptide is known as a gene. To retrieve this information a single-stranded messenger RNA (mRNA) copy of the

gene is made and the sequence of bases in the mRNA is then translated into a linear sequence of amino acids, composing a polypeptide. Genetic information is therefore stored in cells in DNA. During the expression of a gene a segment of DNA is first transcribed into RNA and then translated from RNA into protein. During cell division DNA replicates itself to form two identical DNA helices.

DNA

DNA is composed of three principal components:

1 bases;
2 sugars;
3 phosphates.

These are kept together by three principal types of linkage:

1 covalent bond;
2 hydrogen bond;
3 ester link.

The players

Bases

A base is a molecule that can combine with hydrogen ions in solution. The bases in DNA are nitrogen-containing rings (the nitrogen makes these molecules basic). Pyrimidines (C, T) have one ring, while purines (A, G) have two.

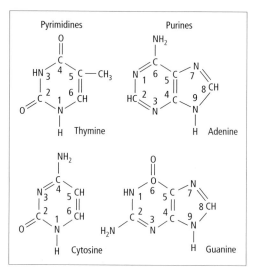

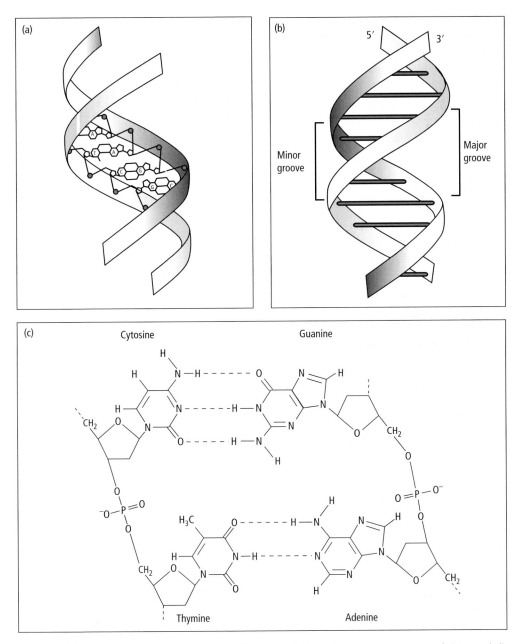

Figure 1.1 (a) Diagrammatic representation of the DNA helix. (b) The major and minor grooves of the DNA helix. (c) CG/TA base pairing.

Sugars

The sugars in DNA are pentoses (sugar molecules containing five carbon atoms). In DNA the pentose is always deoxyribose, indicating that it lacks an oxygen-containing hydroxyl group that is present in ribose,

the parent compound. Ribose could not fit into a DNA helix as there is insufficient room for the 2'-OH group.

By convention the carbon atoms in ribose and deoxyribose are labelled by primed numbers (1' to 5') when part of a nucleotide. This labelling is important in understanding how the DNA molecule is assembled.

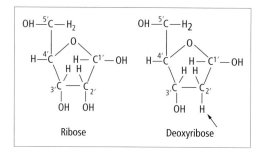

Ribose   Deoxyribose

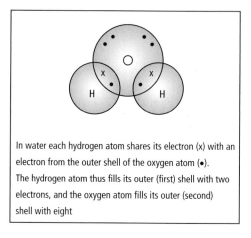

In water each hydrogen atom shares its electron (x) with an electron from the outer shell of the oxygen atom (•). The hydrogen atom thus fills its outer (first) shell with two electrons, and the oxygen atom fills its outer (second) shell with eight

Phosphates

The phosphates in DNA are either mono- or di- or triphosphates. The acidic character of nucleic acid is due to the presence of phosphate esters, which are relatively strong acids (molecules that release a hydrogen ion in solution). At neutral pH they dissociate from hydrogen ions and are thus normally referred to in their ionized form:

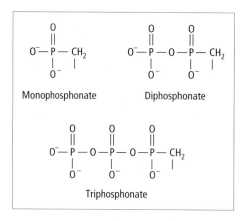

Monophosphonate   Diphosphonate

Triphosphonate

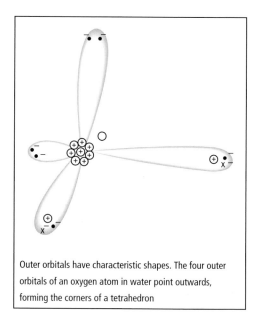

Outer orbitals have characteristic shapes. The four outer orbitals of an oxygen atom in water point outwards, forming the corners of a tetrahedron

The ties that bind

Covalent bonds

A covalent bond exists between atoms that share electrons in their outermost shell. The bonding electrons move freely around both nuclei, which are held close together in a strong bond – energy is released when the bonds are formed, and the same amount of energy is required to break the bond.

Hydrogen bond

A hydrogen atom can usually form only one covalent bond with another atom. A covalently bonded (*electron-depleted*) hydrogen atom can, however, form a weak electrostatic interaction (*hydrogen bond*) with an electronegative (*electron-rich*) atom (usually nitrogen or oxygen), for example,

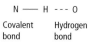

Covalent   Hydrogen
bond   bond

Ester linkage

An ester link involves covalent bonding. It is formed when an alcohol and an acid unite with elimination of water.

Bond Strength

The strength of the bonds is important in understanding the stability of different parts of the final DNA molecule. Strong covalent bonds link nucleic acids in a single DNA strand, whereas weaker hydrogen bonds hold the two complementary DNA strands together.

The formation of DNA

Base + sugar = nucleoside

The 1' carbon of pentose ring is attached to nitrogen 1 of pyrimidine or nitrogen 9 of purine.

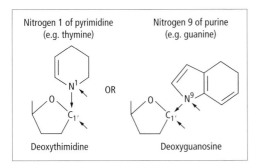

Nitrogen 1 of pyrimidine (e.g. thymine)   Nitrogen 9 of purine (e.g. guanine)

OR

Deoxythimidine   Deoxyguanosine

Base + sugar + phosphate = nucleotide

Phosphate is attached to the 5'-carbon of the pentose ring.

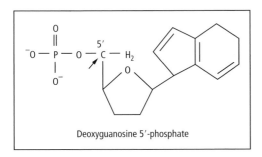

Deoxyguanosine 5'-phosphate

Nucleotides as Energy Stores

Nucleotides may have either one or two or three phosphates attached. In addition to forming the building blocks of DNA, the nucleotide di- and triphosphates are important stores of chemical energy; cleavage of the terminal diphosphate releases energy which is used to drive cell functions. Adenosine triphosphate (ATP) is the most widely used energy carrier in the cell.

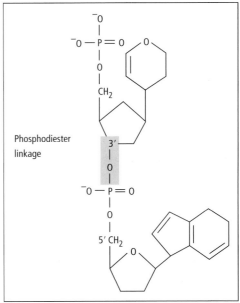

Phosphodiester linkage

Nucleotides join together to form nucleic acid

The hydroxyl group attached to the 3'-pentose carbon of one nucleotide forms an ester link with the phosphate of another molecule, eliminating a water molecule. The link between nucleotides is known as a phosphodiester link.

Thus, one end of a DNA strand has a sugar residue in which the 5'-carbon is not linked to another sugar residue (the 5' end), whereas at the other end the 3'-carbon lacks a phosphodiester link (the 3' end). This simple terminology is fundamental to understanding descriptions of how DNA replicates and is expressed.

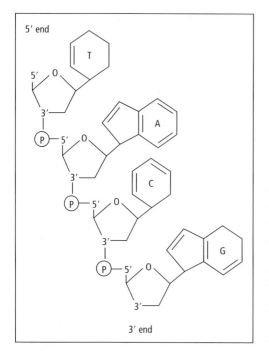

5′ end

3′ end

DNA structure

The DNA helix

In the 1950s X-ray diffraction data suggested that DNA is helical (Figure 1.1(a)). In addition, biochemical data showed that the amount of A in DNA always equalled that of T, whilst the amount of G equalled that of C. These observations led Watson and Crick to propose the double helical structure of DNA, which could account for the physical properties of DNA and its replication in the cell.

The 'backbone' on the outside of the helix consists of alternating sugars and phosphates. The bases are attached to the sugars and form the 'rungs' of the helix.

As the distance between the sugar–phosphate backbone is fixed by the diameter of the helix, only two types of base pairs (bp) (AT or CG) can fit, explaining the constant regularity in the ratios between base pairs (A = T and G = C) (Figure 1.1(c)).

The strands are antiparallel (their 5′,3′-phosphodiester links run in opposite directions) and complementary (because of base pairing the chains complement each other). The sequences of

bases on one strand can thus be deduced from the sequences of bases on the other, and each strand independently carries the information needed to form a double helix.

The DNA helix can take on several conformations. The most common form is *B-DNA*, in which the helix is right handed and has just over 10 bp per helical turn. There are two unequal grooves, the major and minor grooves (Figure 1.1(b)).

A-DNA is a right-handed helix which is shorter and wider than B-DNA. The phosphate groups bind fewer water molecules, and its formation is thus favoured by dehydration. The transition from B-DNA to dehydrated A-DNA was observed during the first X-ray studies of DNA over 50 years ago. The existence of the A-form in many protein–DNA complexes suggests that reversible B–A transition may be important for processing genetic information *in vivo*.

Z-DNA is a left-handed helix in which alternating purines and pyrimidines give rise to a zigzag appearance to the helix. Limited segments of Z-DNA occur *in vivo*. For example, sequences of

Cleavage of DNA Bonds

The relative weakness of the hydrogen bonds holding the complementary bp together is demonstrated by 'melting' the DNA. At increased temperatures the two strands separate: the DNA melts. The bonds holding the backbone of the helix together are stronger and do not melt but can be cleaved by enzymes derived from bacteria, which cut the backbone at specific sites. Bacteria use these enzymes as protective devices to degrade foreign DNA. They restrict the growth of viruses which infect bacteria (bacteriophages) and are known as restriction enzymes. A bacteriophage is a virus that infects bacteria sometimes referred to as a phage.

Describing a DNA Sequence

It is conventional to describe a DNA sequence by writing the sequence of bases in one strand only, and in the 5′ → 3′ direction. When identifying just two neighbouring bases in a sequence it is *usual to insert 'p'* between them to denote an intervening phosphodiester link (e.g. ApT). This is distinct from AT which indicates a hydrogen-bonded base pair on complementary strands.

Z-DNA can be induced at the 5′ ends of genes by transcription, where the Z-form may play a role in RNA processing.

DNA in eukaryotic organisms is organized into a nucleus

Living things may be divided into prokaryotes and eukaryotes. Prokaryotic organisms are simple, single-cell life forms that lack a distinct nucleus. Examples include bacteria and certain algae. Eukaryotes may be single-cell life forms such as yeasts or complex multicellular organisms such as plants and animals. The cells in eukaryotic organisms contain nuclei. DNA within the nucleus of eukaryotes is organized into chromosomes. Each chromosome contains an extensively folded DNA double helix.

Chromatin

The total length of all the strands of DNA in a human cell is ~2 m, all of which needs to be packed into a nucleus a few micrometers in diameter. This is achieved by the formation of a nucleoprotein complex called *chromatin* in which acidic phosphates in the backbone of DNA enable it to form ionic bonds with basic lysine- and arginine-rich proteins known as histones. Coiling of DNA around histone proteins allows long strands to be tightly packed into chromatin.

The core of the nucleosome contains two copies each of histone proteins named H2A, H2B, H3 and H4. A fifth histone, H1, protects the DNA linking the nucleosomes together. Histones can be modified by the addition of an acetyl, methyl or phosphate group in a manner that will alter chromatin structure and function. Variants of these histones encoded by different genes have also been described and shown to be important in functions such as DNA repair.

DNA is first packaged into a *nucleosome* (Figure 1.2), which consists of eight histone proteins around which a strand of DNA containing 146 bp is wound one and three-quarter times.

The histone protein H1 binds to DNA just next to each nucleosome and is involved in coiling DNA into chromatin fibres of 30 nm in diameter (Figure 1.3).

DNA in Prokaryotes

In prokaryotes all the DNA exists in a single molecule, which is circular. There are no 5′ or 3′ ends and no histones and there is no nucleus. The DNA can, however, be induced to supercoil into a compact structure around DNA-binding proteins by the enzyme DNA gyrase.

Chromosomes

During cell division chromatin becomes more condensed and can be recognized in the form of *chromosomes* by light microscopy. During metaphase in mitosis (Figure 1.9) each chromosome consists of two symmetrical *chromatids*, each containing DNA in which the chromatin fibres are folded in loops around a central scaffold of non-histone proteins.

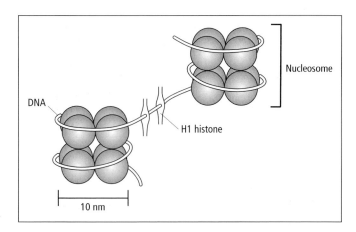

Figure 1.2 A nucleosome.

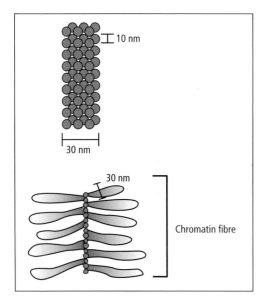

Figure 1.3 A chromatin 30 nm fibre.

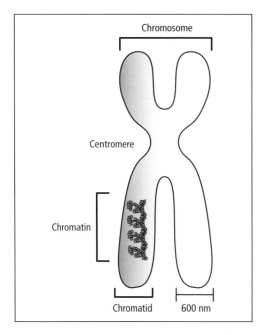

Figure 1.4 Chromosomes, chromatids and chromatin.

The chromatids are attached to each other at the centromere (Figure 1.4).

Condensed metaphase chromosomes can be visualized under the light microscope by various treatments which cause the appearance of light and dark bands. For example, staining with Giemsa gives rise to alternating dark- and pale-staining *G bands* (Figure 1.5). Such banding allows classification of sites on the chromosome according to their location on the short arm (p for petit), or long arm (q), and their position relative to the centromere. For example, the gene that encodes the β-globin chain of haemoglobin (which is abnormal in β thalassaemia), has been localized to the short arm of chromosome 11, in region 1, band 5, sub-band 5: written as 11p15.5 (Figure 1.5).

Chromosome Banding

G-banding with Giemsa stain yields the familiar pattern of ~500 light- and dark-stained bands at metaphase (Figure 1.6); Q-banding with quinacrine, a fluorochrome, yields a fluorescent pattern very similar to that seen in G-banding.

Giemsa developed his staining technique in the early twentieth century. Fluorescent chromosome banding was introduced in 1969 by Caspersson and Zech. The banding patterns of chromosomes from humans, chimpanzees, gorillas and orangutans are remarkably similar.

Euchromatin and Heterochromatin

Euchromatin is genetically active and stains lightly with basic dyes. Heterochromatin is the darker staining condensed region of chromosomes that is characterized by the presence of highly repetitive sequences and relatively low gene density.

Centromeres, Telomeres and Arrays

The *centromere* is the site at which chromosomes constrict during metaphase. It separates the long and short arms of the chromosome.

The *telomere* forms the end of the chromosome.

In *tandemly repeated arrays* identical DNA sequences appear one after the other along a stretch of DNA.

Karyotype

Every species has a specific number and arrangement of chromosomes, which is referred to as a *karyotype*. Human cells contain 46 chromosomes, of which two are sex chromosomes (two X chromosomes in females, an X and a Y chromosome in males), and 44 are autosomes (22 matching pairs numbered 1–22) (Figure 1.6).

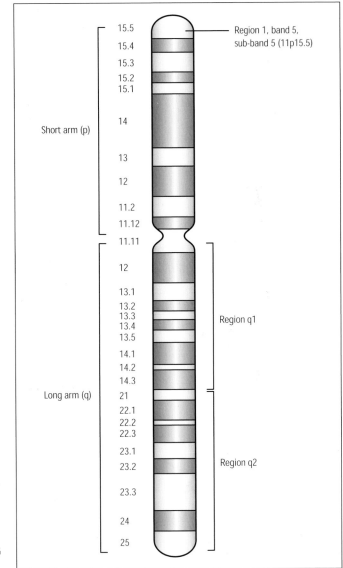

Figure 1.5 Chromosome 11 with G bands.

Genome

The complete genetic make-up of an individual is referred to as their *genome*. Thus, in human cells the genome is composed of 23 pairs of chromosomes within the nucleus, each chromosome containing a single, linear, double-helical strand of DNA. The human genome contains approximately 3×10^9 bp and is thought to contain about 23 000 different genes, most of which encode polypeptides. A small minority of genes encode RNA molecules that are not translated into proteins.

In addition to the nuclear genome, eukaryotic cells also contain a small mitochondrial genome which one tends to inherit from the mother. This is because, unlike sperm, eggs have a considerable amount of cytoplasm which contains mitochondria. In humans the mitochondrial genome consists of a 16 569-bp

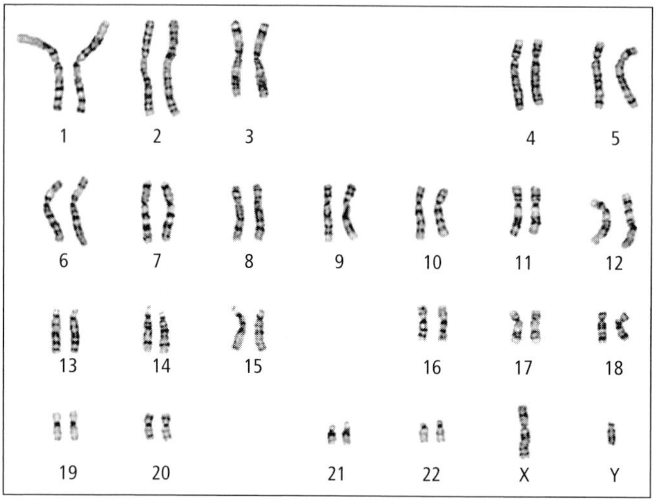

Figure 1.6 A normal human male karyotype stained with Giemsa.

circular DNA molecule which encodes proteins essential for mitochondrial structure and function, including oxidative enzymes, together with RNA molecules involved in mitochondrial protein synthesis (*see* Chapter 2). Although mitochondria possess their own genome, the majority of mitochondrial proteins are encoded by nuclear genes.

DNA replication

The double helical structure of DNA provides a mechanism by which nucleic acids can accurately replicate. Each DNA strand serves as a template for the synthesis of a new complementary strand of DNA. DNA replication is *semiconservative* – one strand (half of the original DNA) is retained ('conserved') in the new DNA molecule.

Much of our understanding of how DNA replicates has come from the study of the bacterium *Escherichia coli*, in which DNA is present as a single circular molecule. Replication starts at a specific site (the origin of replication of the *E. coli* chromosome is termed *oriC*), and proceeds sequentially in opposite directions by formation of discontinuous fragments, which are then joined together by the enzyme DNA ligase. The enzyme polymerase assembles the nucleotides on the new DNA strand and the enzyme exonuclease edits and corrects the process by removing unwanted nucleotides.

During DNA replication the following processes occur (Figure 1.7):

● The double-stranded helix must first unwind and each strand then acts as a template. DNA helicase stimulates separation of the two strands and DNA gyrase aids unwinding. DNA binding proteins then bind to and stabilize the single-stranded structure. This exposes the DNA *template* containing a region of single-stranded DNA from which a complementary copy is made.

● A short strand of RNA, known as a *primer*, is synthesized by an enzyme known as *RNA polymerase* or *Primase* on the DNA template at the start of replication, and removed at the end – *RNA primes the synthesis of DNA*.

● *DNA polymerases* (Pols) catalyse the addition of nucleotides to the primer RNA forming a new strand of DNA. DNA Pols produce a link between the inner phosphorus of the nucleotide and the 3′-OH group of the primer – elongation occurs in the 5′-3′ direction.

● Replication starts at a specific site and proceeds sequentially in opposite directions, even though synthesis can only occur in the 5′-3′ direction. This apparent paradox was resolved by the demonstration that synthesis of one strand occurs continuously, whereas the other strand is synthesized in short 5′ → 3′ fragments, known as Okazaki fragments.

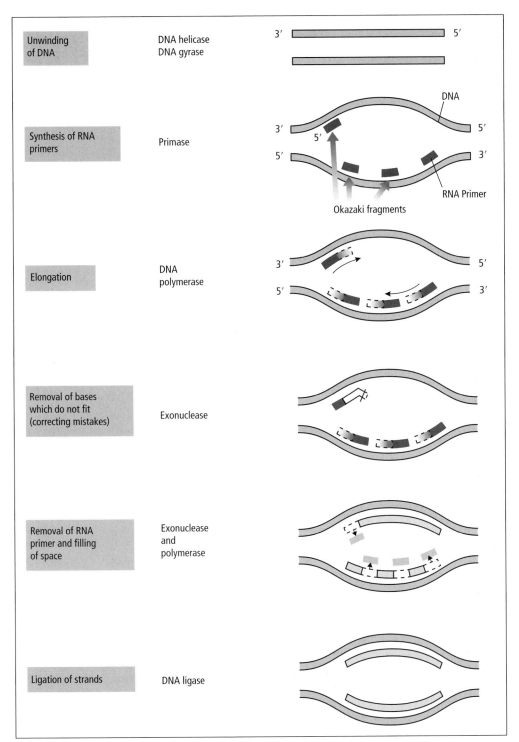

Figure 1.7 Replication of DNA: driving both ways down a one-way street.

• The newly formed DNA is edited by *exonucleases*, enzymes that cut nucleotides from the ends of DNA.
• The RNA primer is removed and the gaps are filled with DNA by a polymerase.
• The Okazaki fragments are joined together by DNA ligase.
• The whole process requires *energy* which is supplied by the hydrolysis of nucleoside triphosphates releasing the diphosphate molecule pyrophosphate. A high-energy phosphoanhydride bond in pyrophosphate is then split, releasing two molecules of inorganic phosphate and providing a source of energy.

DNA Replication

Helicase unwinds part of the double helix
DNA polymerase binds to one strand of the DNA and moves along it in the 3′ to 5′ direction, assembling a leading strand of nucleotides and reforming a double helix.
A different DNA polymerase binds to the other DNA strand and synthesizes discontinuous segments of nucleotides in the 5′ to 3′ direction
DNA ligase joins these together into the lagging strand.

E. coli actually contains three different DNA Pols (I, II and III) which catalyse both the formation and hydrolysis of DNA. The first DNA Pol to be described, DNA Pol I, was found to have the following three different enzymatic activities:
• a polymerase that catalyses the formation of new phosphodiester bonds in the elongating DNA chain;
• a 3′–5′ exonuclease that catalyses the removal of nucleotides from the 3′ end of DNA chains;
• a 5′–3′ exonuclease that cleaves bonds within one chain of a double helix.

The 3′–5′ exonuclease is thought to edit each newly attached base and remove any which are mismatched and will not fit into a double helix. This 'proofreading' activity greatly increases the fidelity of replication. A 5′–3′ exonuclease activity can clear the way ahead for the polymerase activity, digesting the old strand. This activity probably removes the RNA primer that initiates DNA replication and repairs double stranded DNA that is damaged.

Polymerase I can itself be cleaved to yield two fragments: a small fragment containing the 5′–3′ exonuclease, and a large fragment with DNA polymerase and 3′–5′ exonuclease activity.

Most of the DNA in *E. coli* is in fact synthesized by Pol III, whereas repair of the DNA and removal of the RNA primer is predominantly performed by Pol I.

Polymerase Rules

There are many different DNA polymerases, often several in an organism, but they have one activity in common: adding nucleotides (Figure 1.8).
• All polymerases require an end to extend; none can synthesize DNA *de novo*.
• All polymerases extend the 3′-OH end (5′ → 3′ polymerase); no DNA Pol adds to the 5′ end.
• Nearly all polymerases make a reverse copy (the *complement*) of the template strand.
The last rule is not absolute because there *are* enzymes that polymerize DNA and work without a template strand, but these are used relatively infrequently (e.g. terminal deoxytransferase (TdT), which adds a 'tail' of nucleotides). The first two rules of DNA Pols might make you think again about how genomic DNA is replicated. DNA Pol cannot start synthesizing DNA *de novo*, so instead replication of genomic DNA starts with RNA primers of ~10 bp length, which are first extended and then replaced with DNA by DNA Pol. Both strands are replicated as the 'replication fork' moves in one direction. Replication in the 5′–3′ direction is easy because that is the direction of DNA polymerization. In the 3′–5′ direction, small pieces of DNA (1000–2000 bp) are synthesized in the 5′–3′ direction and then ligated together.

Many DNA polymerases also possess exonuclease activities.

Nuclease Anarchy

Nucleases cut nucleic acids either into big pieces (*endonucleases*) or many little pieces (*exonucleases*). Exonucleases can be seen as undoing the work of polymerases: they depolymerize. Unlike the relatively uniform world of polymerases, however, nucleases demonstrate a wide range of abilities.
• Some exonucleases chew from one end (5′ → 3′).
• Some exonucleases chew from the other end (3′ → 5′).
• Some *endo*nucleases take a bite right out of the middle, not starting at an end.

DNA replication in eukaryotic cells

A similar mechanism for DNA replication occurs in eukaryotic cells, although the process differs in the following respects.
• Polymerases in eukaryotic cells include polymerase a, b, d (located in the nucleus) and g (located in mitochondria).
• Because of the size of eukaryotic genomes replication originates at many sites within each chromosome.
• In prokaryotic cells the two daughter chromosomes segregate and the cell divides as soon as the chromosome has duplicated. In eukaryotic cells DNA synthesis and cell division occur at different times.

The whole process of cell growth and division in eukaryotic cells can be divided into different phases, which together make up the cell cycle.

Eukaryotic cell cycle

The eukaryotic cell cycle (Figure 1.9) consists of two periods: (1) the M (mitotic) period (Figure 1.10) during which cell division occurs; and (2) interphase during which cell growth and DNA replication occur. Interphase is further divided into:
• G1 (gap 1);
• S (synthetic);
• G2 (gap 2) phases.

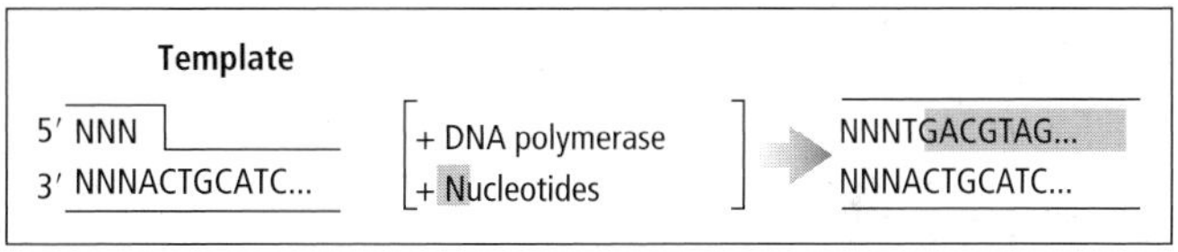

Figure 1.8 DNA polymerases add to the 3′ end of the DNA nucleotides that match the opposite strand, the template.

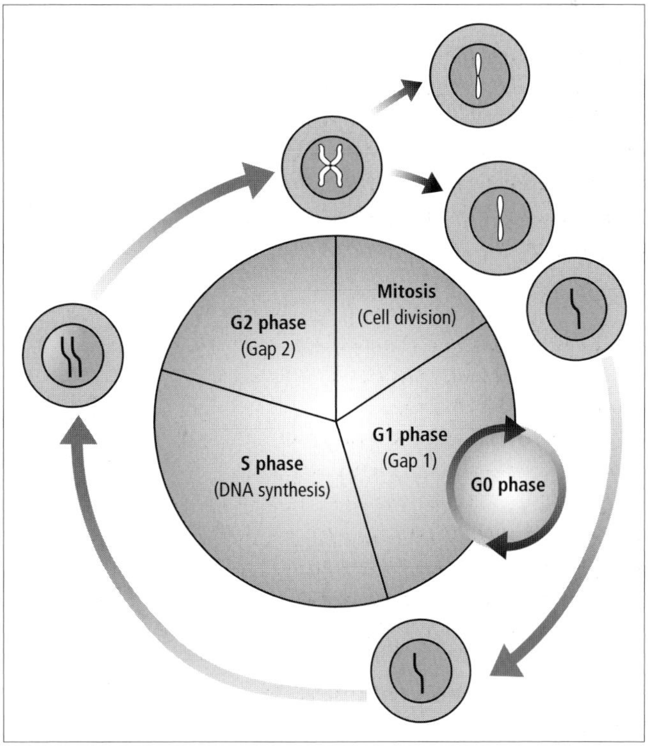

Figure 1.9 Eukaryotic cell cycle.

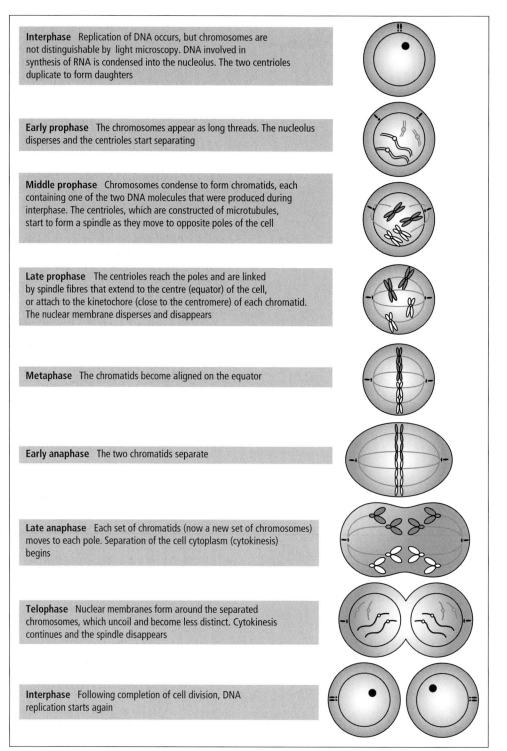

Interphase Replication of DNA occurs, but chromosomes are not distinguishable by light microscopy. DNA involved in synthesis of RNA is condensed into the nucleolus. The two centrioles duplicate to form daughters

Early prophase The chromosomes appear as long threads. The nucleolus disperses and the centrioles start separating

Middle prophase Chromosomes condense to form chromatids, each containing one of the two DNA molecules that were produced during interphase. The centrioles, which are constructed of microtubules, start to form a spindle as they move to opposite poles of the cell

Late prophase The centrioles reach the poles and are linked by spindle fibres that extend to the centre (equator) of the cell, or attach to the kinetochore (close to the centromere) of each chromatid. The nuclear membrane disperses and disappears

Metaphase The chromatids become aligned on the equator

Early anaphase The two chromatids separate

Late anaphase Each set of chromatids (now a new set of chromosomes) moves to each pole. Separation of the cell cytoplasm (cytokinesis) begins

Telophase Nuclear membranes form around the separated chromosomes, which uncoil and become less distinct. Cytokinesis continues and the spindle disappears

Interphase Following completion of cell division, DNA replication starts again

Figure 1.10 Mitosis.

DNA synthesis occurs only during the S phase of the cell cycle, which is followed by a gap period (G2) before cell division (mitosis) occurs. Mitosis is followed by a further gap period (G1) during which the cell prepares for DNA synthesis. Cells which are not preparing for DNA synthesis and cell division may leave G1 and enter a stage called G0. Such cells may be metabolically active, but they do not proceed through the cell cycle. G0 may represent a temporary quiescent state, from which the cell returns to G1 or a terminally differentiated state. Non-replicating cells such as nerve cells are generally stopped in G0.

The vast majority of the cells of the body are non-replicating. Skin cells, intestinal epithelium, haematopoietic bone marrow cells and a few other cell types replicate throughout life.

Mitosis

Mitosis is a process of cell division during which two daughter cells are produced from a single parent cell. The daughter cells are identical to one another and to the original parent cell. Each daughter cell must receive a share of all of the organelles (*see* Figure 1.23) such as mitochondria, ribosomes, lysosomes, endoplasmic reticulum, Golgi body and centrioles (*see* Box "Centrosome", above), together with two complete genomes, which make a complete set of genes. Ensuring that each daughter cell receives two copies of every gene requires great precision.

Mitosis allows the equal partitioning of replicated chromosomes into two identical groups. Before partitioning of chromosomes that have replicated during interphase occurs, the chromosomes become aligned so that they can separate in an orderly fashion. To do this the chromosomes interact with hollow tubular filaments known as microtubules, which become organized into a spindle and then pull the chromosomes apart. During the interphase before mitosis the centrioles and other components of the centrosome are duplicated, but remain together as a single structure. At the beginning of mitosis the centrosome splits and the two centrosomes move apart until they are on opposite sides of the nucleus. As mitosis proceeds microtubules grow out from each centrosome to create the clusters of microtubules, which form spindle fibres. At the same time chromatin begins to coil and supercoil making it more compact and chromosomes condense to form identical paired chromatids of chromosomes. The nuclear envelope breaks down and the spindle microtubules become attached to the centromere of chromosomes through a structure known as the kinetochore. The centromere regions become aligned at the cell's equator and the centromere divides and the new chromosomes, each derived from one of the paired chromatids, move towards different poles.

Centrosome

Centrioles are paired structures which organize the spindle on which chromosomes are pulled apart in animal cells. The centrosome is a mass of protein also called the microtubule organizing centre (MTOC), which surrounds centrioles. During mitosis, animal cells inherit a single centrosome that contains a pair of centrioles. The younger 'daughter' centriole, which was formed during the previous S phase, and the older 'mother' centriole differ structurally from each other.

The process of mitosis can be divided into four stages of prophase, metaphase, anaphase and telophase (Figure 1.10). At the end of mitosis daughter cells separate from each other through a process known as cytokinesis, which differs between animal and plant cells as a consequence of having or not having a cell wall.

Meiosis, the cell division that occurs when mature eggs and sperm are formed, which halves the chromosome number, is described on page 48.

Gene expression: making proteins

A gene is a sequence of DNA which codes for one polypeptide. Transcription is the synthesis of mRNA using the information contained in DNA. Translation is the use of this information to synthesize protein. Gene expression involves the transcription of a segment of DNA into RNA, and the translation of RNA into a polypeptide.

During replication each DNA strand serves as a template for the synthesis of a new complementary strand of DNA, whereas during gene expression information is retrieved from only one of the two available strands. The sense strand of DNA has the same sequence of bases as the transcribed mRNA (in which U (uracil) replaces T). The antisense strand carries the complementary sequence of bases.

The segment of DNA containing a gene is first transcribed into a single-stranded mRNA copy which has the same sequence of bases as the sense strand of DNA and is complementary to the antisense strand. The sequence of bases is then translated into a sequence of amino acids composing a polypeptide. The direction of synthesis of DNA during replication or RNA during transcription is $5' \rightarrow 3'$.

The flow of genetic information can thus be summarized as follows:

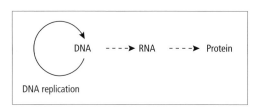

DNA replication

Genetic information can also pass from RNA to RNA during replication of some RNA viruses and from RNA to DNA in retroviruses, which have RNA genomes from which a DNA copy is made during their infectious cycle.

Viruses
Viruses are small, intracellular parasites which generally consist of DNA or RNA within a protein coat or capsid. In some complex viruses a membrane surrounds the protein coat. A virus cannot replicate by itself, but uses the machinery of infected cells to do so.

The retrovirus genome contains the gene for the enzyme reverse transcriptase which catalyses RNA-dependent synthesis of DNA (Figure 1.11).

Genes carry the code for the amino acids in polypeptide chains. The genetic code is the same in all organisms.

The genetic code

The 20 amino acids [alanine (Ala), arginine (Arg), asparagine (Asn), aspartic acid (Asp), cysteine (Cys), glutamine (Gln), glutamic acid (Glu), glycine (Gly), histidine (His), isoleucine (Ile), leucine (Leu), lysine (Lys), methionine (Met), phenylalanine (Phe), proline (Pro), serine (Ser), threonine (Thr), tryptophan (Trp), tyrosine (Tyr) and valine (Val)] are encoded by base triplets. UAA, UAG and UGA cause termination of transcription.

Genetic Coding
Each of the 20 amino acids (for abbreviations *see* p16) is encoded by a triplet of bases (*codon*). Since there are four bases there are $4 \times 4 \times 4 = 64$ possible codons, and single amino acids may be encoded by more than one codon (there is 'redundancy' in the code).
Certain codons specify the beginning and end of polypeptide chains. Methionine, encoded by AUG (or more rarely GAG, which usually encodes valine), is found at the start of polypeptide chains, whereas UAA, UAG and UGA do not specify amino acids, but indicate termination or stop signals at the end of chains.

RNA structure

RNA differs from DNA in the following respects:
- RNA is single stranded (usually).
- The sugar in RNA is ribose rather than deoxyribose.

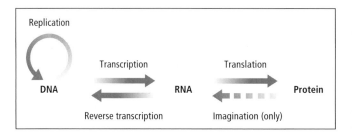

Figure 1.11 The enzyme reverse transcriptase generates complementary DNA from RNA. Reverse translation if it were ever observed could not be precise due to the degeneracy of the genetic code (meaning that nearly every amino acid can be encoded by two or more triplet nucleotide codons).

- RNA has U rather than T as one of its pyrimidines. RNA exists in several forms. Only messenger RNA (mRNA) is formed as a copy of a gene encoding a specific polypeptide. Small non-translated RNA molecules perform many functions in relation to gene expression and are formed as the products of genes which actually encode RNA molecules.
- *mRNA* is a copy of DNA which encodes a specific amino acid sequence.
- *Transfer RNA (tRNA)* carries amino acids to ribosomes.
- *Ribosomal RNA (rRNA)* facilitates the interaction between mRNA and tRNA, resulting in the translation of mRNA into protein.
- *Small nuclear RNA* is involved in RNA splicing, a process by which non-coding sequences are cut out of mRNA.
- *Small nucleolar RNA* modifies ribosomal RNA.

Ribosomes

The code carried by mRNA is read and translated into protein in ribosomes. Ribosomes are structures found in the cytoplasm of cells composed of rRNA and proteins. A triplet codon on mRNA is matched by an anticodon on tRNA, which holds the correct amino acid. Peptide bonds form between the amino acids, creating a polypeptide chain (see Figure 1.20).

---

tRNA and rRNA

tRNA molecules differ according to the amino acid they carry. About 1600 copies of genes encoding different tRNA molecules are dispersed throughout the human genome.

rRNA is formed of different-sized subunits, designated 28S, 5.8S, 18S and 5S. The 28S, 5.8S and 18S subunits are formed by processing a large precursor RNA molecule encoded by about 300 copies of a gene which occurs on chromosomes 13, 14, 15, 21 and 22. Copies of the gene encoding the 5S subunit are clustered together on chromosome 1.

Subunits of RNA are commonly designated S, or Svedberg units, which are related to the size and shape of the RNA. Svedberg units are actually measures of the sedimentation rate of molecules centrifuged through a density gradient. This was a common method of analysing macromolecules before gel electrophoresis (see p 31) became routine.

- *Small interfering RNA (siRNA)* mediate RNA interference, a process by which mRNA is degraded.
- *Micro RNA (miRNA)* prevents translation of mRNA.

Gene transcription: transmitting the code

RNA transcription can be divided into stages of:
- initiation;
- elongation;
- termination.

As with DNA replication, the process of gene transcription is more fully understood in prokaryotic than in eukaryotic organisms. This in part reflects the simpler nature of prokaryotic genomes, which consist of closely packed genes, in which the coding DNA sequences are rarely interrupted.

Prokaryotic gene transcription

RNA polymerases make RNA from a DNA template (transcription).

Gene transcription in prokaryotic cells (Figure 1.12) is relatively simple.
- *Initiation*. RNA Pol binds to a specific sequence, known as a promoter, which lies just upstream of the coding sequence of the gene.
- *Elongation*. RNA Pol then proceeds through the gene, synthesizing a RNA chain which is a copy of the antisense strand of DNA. The reaction is similar to the polymerization of DNA (see p 12, especially Boxes "DNA Replication" and "Polymerases Rule"), in that nucleotide triphosphates are hydrolysed releasing pyrophosphate which is split into inorganic phosphate.
- *Termination*. When the polymerase encounters a specific sequence, known as a terminator, transcription stops and the completed RNA molecule is released.

Gene structure and transcription in eukaryotic cells

Differences in both gene structure and the RNA Pol molecules make transcription in eukaryotes more complex.

17

Possible codons of an amino acid

First position	Second position	Third position							
		U		**C**		**A**		**G**	
U	U	F Phenylalanine	Phe	F Phenylalanine	Phe	L Leucine	Leu	L Leucine	Leu
	C	L Leucine	Leu	L Leucine	Leu	L Leucine	Leu	L Leucine	Leu
	A	I Isoleucine	Ile	I Isoleucine	Ile	I Isoleucine	Ile	M Methionine	Met
	G	V Valine	Val	V Valine	Val	V Valine	Val	V Valine	Val
C	U	S Serine	Ser	S Serine	Ser	S Serine	Ser	S Serine	Ser
	C	P Proline	Pro	P Proline	Pro	P Proline	Pro	P Proline	Pro
	A	T Threonine	Thr	T Threonine	Thr	T Threonine	Thr	T Threonine	Thr
	G	A Alanine	Ala	A Alanine	Ala	A Alanine	Ala	A Alanine	Ala
A	U	Y Tyrosine	Tyr	Y Tyrosine	Tyr	– Termination	Stop	– Termination	Stop
	C	H Histidine	His	H Histidine	His	Q Glutamine	Gln	Q Glutamine	Gln
	A	N Asparagine	Asn	N Asparagine	Asn	K Lysine	Lys	K Lysine	Lys
	G	D Aspartic Acid	Asp	D Aspartic Acid	Asp	E Glutamate	Glu	E Glutamate	Glu
G	U	C Cysteine	Cys	C Cysteine	Cys	– Termination	Stop	W Tryptophane	Trp
	C	R Argenine	Arg	R Argenine	Arg	R Argenine	Arg	R Argenine	Arg
	A	S Serine	Ser	S Serine	Ser	R Argenine	Arg	R Argenine	Arg
	G	G Glycine	Gly	G Glycine	Gly	G Glycine	Gly	G Glycine	Gly

Each amino acid has a one letter code (top left corner of each column) and three letter code (top right hand corner of each column), and is encoded by more than one codon.

There are three RNA polymerases, transcription is regulated by numerous different proteins, most of which bind to specific sites around the coding region of the gene, and mRNA is modified in several ways before being ready for translation into protein.

• RNA Pol I transcribes the rRNA genes.

• RNA Pol II transcribes the protein-coding genes, making mRNA.

• RNA Pol III transcribes the tRNA genes.

Pol II is the most intensively studied because of its role in gene and protein expression. Gene expression is often regulated by the rate of transcription, which is largely controlled by the binding of RNA

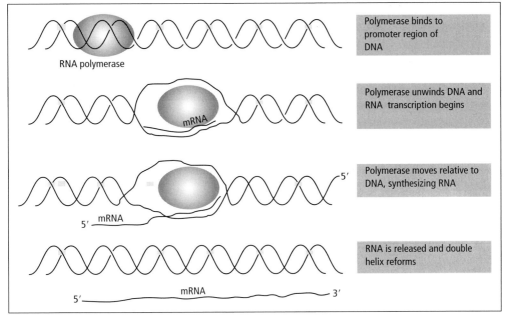

Figure 1.12 Transcription in prokaryotes.

Within the figure:

- RNA polymerase
- Polymerase binds to promoter region of DNA
- mRNA
- Polymerase unwinds DNA and RNA transcription begins
- 5′
- 5′ mRNA
- Polymerase moves relative to DNA, synthesizing RNA
- RNA is released and double helix reforms
- 5′ — mRNA — 3′

Pol II to the gene promoter. Since RNA Pol II must transcribe many different genes, it is helped to identify exactly *which* gene should be transcribed and *when* by gene-specific proteins. These proteins bind to sequences in the gene, called enhancers or silencers, that act to increase or decrease transcription. Additional proteins help RNA Pol II to find exactly the correct start (initiation) and end (termination).

Reading the Helical DNA Template

It is not known exactly how RNA polymerase manages to read the helical DNA template, analogous to reading an inscription circling round a column, without getting the ever lengthening RNA transcript hopelessly tangled. It is likely that the DNA is nicked and then rotates around the (other) single strand beneath the RNA polymerase. One reason this is thought to be true is because in bacteria the RNA message is already being translated before transcription is complete and it seems improbable that the whole RNA polymerase–mRNA–ribosome complex could spin around the DNA. Although RNA polymerase is fast (bacterial RNA polymerase adds 60 nucleotides/s), at this rate it takes nearly an *hour* to transcribe the 186 000-bp gene encoding the human clotting factor VII.

Only a small fraction of the human genome encodes polypeptides; over 95% is non-coding with no known function. Non-coding DNA occurs both within and between genes. Some of this apparently functionless DNA contains repetitive sequences of bases, which may be of functional significance. For example, centromeres which ensure complete disjunction at the middle of chromosomes, and telomeres which allow complete replication at the ends of chromosomes, both contain arrays of tandemly repeated DNA.

The structure of eukaryotic genes is more complex than a series of codons. The transcriptional unit of a gene is the region transcribed into a primary RNA transcript, which is a precursor of mRNA. It is made up of *exons* (containing *expressed* or coding DNA), which are interrupted by sequences of unknown function known as *intervening sequences* (IVS) or *introns* (Figure 1.13). Introns begin with GT and end with AG.

The coding regions in the first and last exons are flanked by untranslated regions (UTRs), which are actually part of the exons and are transcribed into mRNA but not translated into protein.

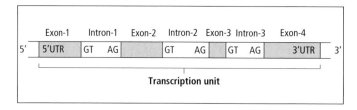

Figure 1.13 Diagrammatic representation of a eukaryotic transcription unit. UTR, untranslated region.

Transcription and Control Regions

The promoter region is located immediately upstream of the gene-coding region and contains sequences that govern the rate of transcription and define the site at which it starts.

Enhancer/silencer regions may be located within, near or some distance away from the gene whose expression they stimulate/suppress.

Structures which facilitate the binding of proteins to DNA have been identified. For example, *zinc fingers* consist of a fold of about 30 amino acids around a zinc atom, which seems to insert into grooves in the DNA helix. *Leucine zippers* contain four or five leucine residues, each one spaced exactly seven residues apart. Pairs of DNA-binding proteins can attach to each other along the 'zipper', and the whole structure then appears to grip the DNA helix, bringing the DNA-binding proteins into contact with their binding domains.

Sequences on the 5' side of a region of DNA (to the left in a 5'–3' sequence) are often called 'upstream', whereas those on the 3' side are 'downstream'.

DNA sequences that influence the transcription of genes are known as *cis-acting control elements*. They do not encode proteins, but often influence gene transcription by acting as binding sites for protein produced by other genes, known as *trans-acting transcription factors* or *DNA-binding proteins*. These DNA-binding proteins may influence gene transcription by altering DNA to expose or hide certain sequences or changes in the position of DNA with respect to the nuclear membrane.

cis-acting control regions are usually organized in clusters, which are located in the *promoter* and *enhancer* regions of the gene.

Certain DNA sequences are found in the *promoter region* of most genes (Figure 1.14). These include the TATA and CAAT boxes.

• *TATA box.* Consists of an AT-rich sequence (often TATAA) which occurs about 30 bp upstream from the transcriptional start site (often denoted −30: the position of the nucleotide at the start site is designated +1). TATA boxes are often absent from the promoters of 'housekeeping genes'. Housekeeping genes, such as genes encoding the structural protein actin, are continuously expressed at low levels and often have GC-rich sequences such as GGGCGG in their promoter regions.

• *CAAT box.* Contains this short sequence about 80 bp upstream (−80) of the start site.

These sequences, together with binding sites for other transcription factors which vary according to the gene involved, are responsible for the rate of transcription (Figure 1.15).

Transcription starts at the *CAP site*, so called because following transcription, the 5' end of the

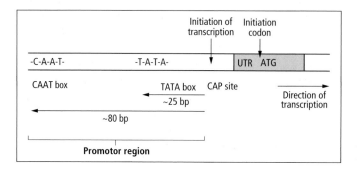

Figure 1.14 The promoter region is a short nucleotide sequence at the 5' end of a gene, just upstream of the transcription start site. In addition to a CAAT box and TATA box, sequences within the promoter region and often some distance away bind enhancers and silencers that increase or decrease transcription of a gene.

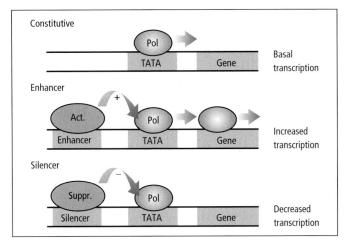

Figure 1.15 Constitutive transcription is the basal rate of gene transcription. Different genes are transcribed constitutively at different rates. An enhancer is a DNA sequence that binds protein activators and increases transcription of a specific gene. A silencer is a DNA sequence that binds repressors and decreases transcription of a specific gene. When transcription increases, RNA polymerases initiate transcription more often but they move down the gene (transcribe) at the same speed.

mRNA is capped at this site by the attachment of a specialized nucleotide (7-methyl guanosine). The cap site is followed by a *leader sequence* leading up to the *initiation codon* (ATG), that specifies the start of translation.

Transcription then proceeds, such that a full copy of the gene (*introns* and *exons*) is made using a process similar to DNA replication (Figure 1.16).

A *stop codon* (TAA, TAG or TGA) does not code for an amino acid and thus signals the end of protein synthesis (Figure 1.17).

This is followed by a UTR, which includes the *poly(A) signal* (AATAAA), that signals cleavage of the newly formed RNA at a position slightly downstream, and the addition of a string of adenylate residues (a poly(A) tail). The poly(A) tail is thus not encoded by the gene; rather adenosine monophosphate residues are sequentially added enzymatically following transcription.

Thus, each end of the mRNA contains a UTR which is not translated into protein. The function of these regions is not fully understood, although the 5′ region (upstream) appears to influence translation, whereas the 3′ region (downstream) may contain sequences that are important in the stability of mRNA.

The 5′ cap binds to the small subunit of the ribosome as the first step in translation.

In eukaryotic cells, transcription is mostly controlled at the level of initiation. The binding of transcription factors to the promoter region of a gene attracts RNA Pol. Three types of RNA Pol (I, II and III) occur in eukaryotes, of which RNA Pol II is principally involved in transcription of mRNA. The primary RNA transcripts produced by RNA Pol II are referred to as *heterogeneous nuclear RNA* (*hnRNA*), because unlike tRNA and rRNA, they show considerable variability (heterogeneity) in size.

The presence of proteins which act as transcription factors is required before a RNA Pol II molecule can recognize and bind to the promoter of a gene and start transcription. These are referred to using the prefix TFII (e.g. TFIIA, TFIIB, TFIID, TFIIE, TFIIF, TFIIH in order of their discovery) because they each act as *transcription factors* for RNA Pol II. TFIID binds to the TATA box and is also known as the TATA factor.

Binding of RNA Pol II to the promoter region of a gene results in a localized separation of double-stranded DNA. During formation of an mRNA molecule about 20 bp of DNA are unwound at any one time, of which around 10 form a DNA/RNA hybrid. The RNA Pol proceeds through the gene and synthesizes an mRNA chain from the 5′ to 3′ end by adding ribonucleoside monophosphate bases complementary to the DNA. Only one strand (the antisense strand) is used as a template. The primary RNA transcript is thus an exact copy of the sense DNA strand, except that U replaces T.

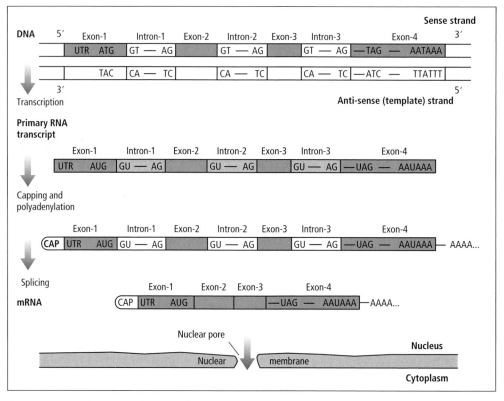

Figure 1.16 Transcription in a eukaryotic cell.

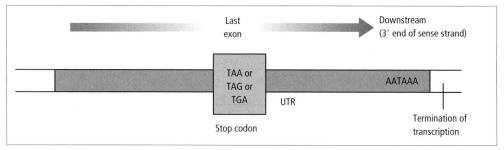

Figure 1.17 Termination of eukaryotic transcription.

Most rRNA is transcribed by RNA Pol I in the nucleolus, whereas the small (5S) rRNA and tRNA are transcribed by RNA Pol III in the extranucleolar region.

Post-transcriptional processing

While still in the nucleus the newly synthesized RNA is modified by the following events:

● *Capping* – the addition of a nucleotide cap.

● *Polyadenylation* – detachment of the RNA and addition of a string of adenosine residues.

● *Splicing* – sequences corresponding to *introns* are *excised* and discarded and the remaining *exons* are *spliced together*.

During splicing all of the introns are usually removed, leaving all of the exons in the mRNA. However, exons may also be removed during the splicing process, resulting in variations in the final mRNA product, and hence in the polypeptide it encodes. The process by which different mRNA transcripts are formed by removal of different segments of the primary RNA transcript is known as alternative splicing (Figure 1.18).

After capping, polyadenylation and splicing, the RNA is then ready for transport to the cytoplasm.

Translation: reading the code

Protein synthesis occurs on ribosomes. In eukaryotes, ribosomes consist of 40S (small) and 60S (large) subunits, which together form 80S particles (S = Svedberg units, *see* p 19). 60S subunits contain proteins complexed to three rRNAs (28S, 5.8S and 5S), whereas in the 40S subunits proteins are complexed to 18S RNA.

The structure of the 30S (small) and 50S (large) subunits of bacterial ribosomes have been resolved at an atomic level. The 30S subunit contains the mRNA decoding site. There are three binding sites for RNA (Figure 1.19).

These are the A (acceptor), P (peptidyl) and E (exit) sites. These three sites are involved in the selection of tRNA, the addition of the amino acid it carries to the growing amino acid chain and the completion of polypeptide synthesis (Figure 1.20).

The process of protein synthesis is started by the formation of a complex involving the small ribosomal subunit carrying a methionine tRNA, which

base pairs with the initiation codon AUG on mRNA (Figure 1.16). Once the initiation complex has formed, synthesis of the polypeptide chain is driven by elongation factors (elFs), which join the large subunit to the complex and move the ribosome relative to the mRNA. Each tRNA carries an amino acid and a triplet of bases (*anticodon*),

which recognize a codon on mRNA specific for the amino acid. For example, the tRNA that carries methionine has the anticodon UAC which recognizes the methionine codon AUG on mRNA. The peptidyl transferase reaction that joins amino acids together is catalysed by RNA molecules which are exposed on the surface of the ribosome by the folded structure it adopts. Thus the ribosome is a ribozyme.

Ribozymes

Some RNA molecules are able to function as enzymes. These catalytic RNA molecules are known as ribozymes. They were initially identified by their ability to cleave RNA.

The ribosome contains RNA molecules that catalyse the formation of peptide bonds that join amino acids during protein synthesis.

When the ribosome reaches a termination codon (UAA, UAG or UGA) the completed polypeptide is released from the last tRNA, and the ribosomal units fall off the mRNA.

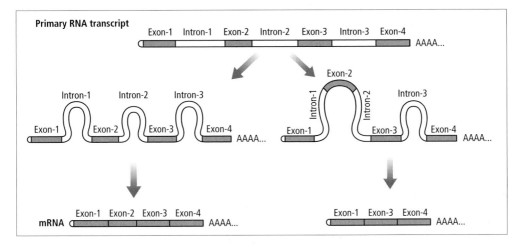

Figure 1.18 Alternative splicing produces different mRNAs from the same primary transcript.

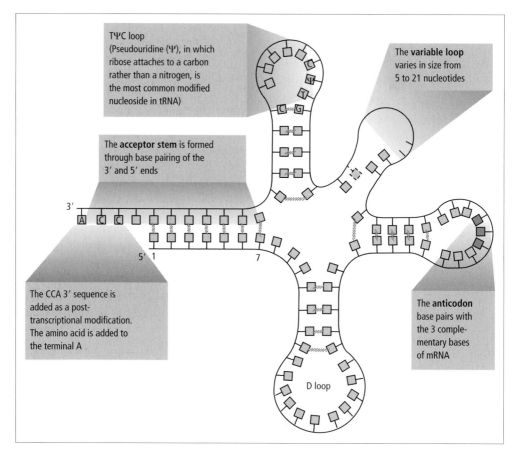

TΨC loop
(Pseudouridine (Ψ), in which ribose attaches to a carbon rather than a nitrogen, is the most common modified nucleoside in tRNA)

The **variable loop** varies in size from 5 to 21 nucleotides

The **acceptor stem** is formed through base pairing of the 3′ and 5′ ends

The CCA 3′ sequence is added as a post-transcriptional modification. The amino acid is added to the terminal A

The **anticodon** base pairs with the 3 complementary bases of mRNA

D loop

Figure 1.19 The structure of tRNA.

Self-regulation: RNA silencing itself

RNA interference – kill the messenger

Double-stranded RNA can *silence* homologous genes through RNA interference (RNAi), a process through which dsRNA (double-stranded RNA) molecules silence gene expression in a sequence specific manner. It probably exists as a protection from viral infection and to modulate transposon activity (p 45).

RNAi involves the processing of large dsRNA molecules into small 21–23 nucleotide siRNA molecules by an enzyme of the RNase III family of nucleases named Dicer. The siRNAs are recruited to a multi-protein complex with RNase activity known as RNA-induced silencing complex (RISC). The siRNA duplex unwinds and an active form of RISC associated only with the antisense strand of siRNA is guided to its complementary target mRNA molecule, which is degraded (Figure 1.21).

RNAi is a powerful means of studying gene function, providing an alternative to creating knockout phenotypes (Chapter 2, p 82), and has attracted considerable interest as a therapeutic tool.

Micro RNAs

miRNA are evolutionary conserved, naturally occurring, non-coding small RNA molecules that regulate post-transcriptional gene expression. One of the first miRNAs to be described was *let-7* (Figure 1.22), which regulates the timing of gene expression during development of the nematode *Caenorhabditis elegans*. *let-7* is highly conserved

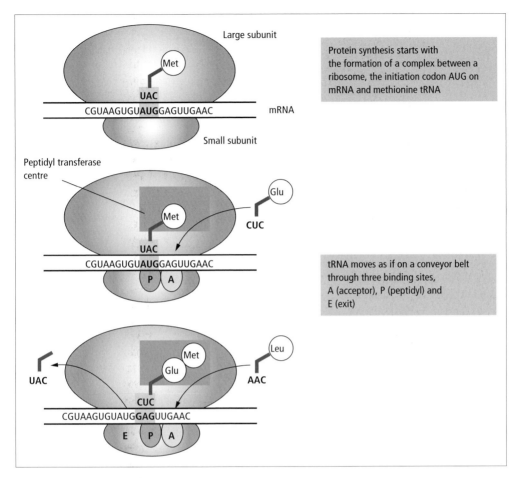

Figure 1.20 Translating the genetic code of mRNA into the polypeptide chain of a protein.

Protein synthesis starts with the formation of a complex between a ribosome, the initiation codon AUG on mRNA and methionine tRNA

tRNA moves as if on a conveyor belt through three binding sites, A (acceptor), P (peptidyl) and E (exit)

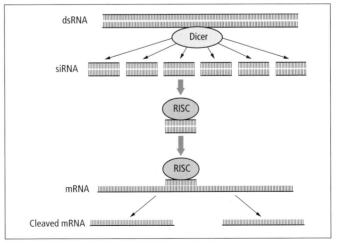

Figure 1.21 RNA interference. dsRNA is recognized by the enzyme complex Dicer and cleaved to siRNAs. siRNA binds to and activates the RNA induced silencing complex (RISC), leading to unwinding of the siRNA. One strand of the siRNA guides the RISC to the target mRNA, which is cleaved preventing protein synthesis.

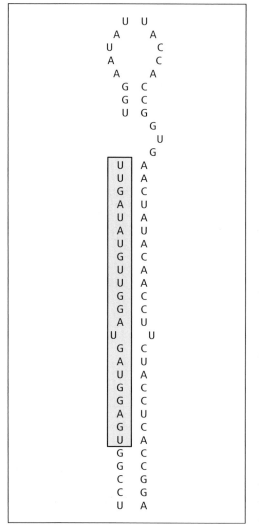

Figure 1.22 A molecular timer: *let-7* in *C. elegans* is thought to be transcribed as a hairpin structure from which the 21 nucleotide mature form (shaded) is processed. Homologous *let-7* genes have been identified in many other species, including humans.

even in humans, and it is now realized that a wide range of miRNA molecules are involved in gene regulation in all species.

Post-translational processing

Polypeptides may start to form the complex structure of proteins as they are synthesized. Secretory proteins pass through the rough endoplasmic reticulum and move to the Golgi body for processing (Figure 1.23). Following synthesis many polypeptides are modified further, for example by hydroxylation or phosphorylation of amino acids, or addition of sugars (glycosylation).

Manipulating DNA and RNA in the laboratory

The fact that genes are composed of only four biochemically similar nucleic acids, which convey information in their sequence and not in their 3-dimensional shape (tertiary structure), makes the chemistry of isolation and characterization correspondingly uniform and largely independent of their sequence.

Nucleic acid preparation and analysis

The relative structural simplicity and homogeneity of nucleic acids led some early researchers to doubt that DNA *could* be the 'stuff' of which genes are made. Nucleic acids were wrongly thought to be merely structural elements of chromosomes, perhaps organizing the proteins that were deemed complicated enough to constitute genes. This reluctance may be harder for us to understand now that so much information is stored digitally in an even simpler binary code.

The trick in preparing nucleic acids is to isolate DNA or RNA from other cellular constituents, without exposing them to enzymes or conditions that will destroy them. Nucleic acids are uniformly and strongly negatively charged because of their phosphate backbones (*see* Box "Basic DNA Structure", p 2). Therefore, they prefer an aqueous (watery) environment where these charges are hydrated instead of an organic (oily) environment. Other cellular constituents, such as proteins, lipids and carbohydrates, contain uncharged as well as charged regions, which make these molecules prefer either an organic environment or the interface between organic and aqueous phases. This is the basis of extraction by the organic solvent phenol and other separations. Nucleic acids are also relatively dense due in part to their heavy phosphate atoms and can therefore be separated on caesium chloride (CsCl) gradients.

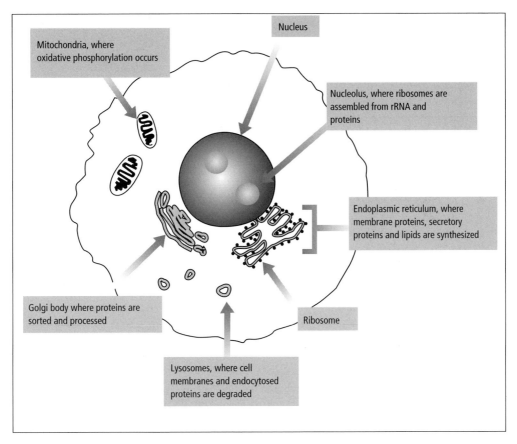

Figure 1.23 Representation of a eukaryotic cell showing some of the important organelles.

The ways in which DNA and RNA *differ*, and how these differences are exploited in their purification, is described next, before embarking on a discussion of their manipulation.

DNA is relatively easy to prepare and store, principally because although DNA-specific degrading enzymes (DNases) are normally abundant they are easily destroyed by moderate heating (65°C). For some purposes, such as preparing single stranded DNA as a template for the polymerase chain reaction (PCR, *see* p 34), it is sufficient simply to lyse the cells (i.e. destroy the cells through rupture of the plasma membrane) and denature the proteins and DNA at high temperature (95°C).

RNA preparation

RNA is prepared most often to analyse gene activity, which is determined by counting the number of mRNA gene transcripts. This can provide information about the level of gene activity during fetal development, during disease states, and in response to treatment. RNA is also prepared to analyse transcript forms (alternative splicing – p 22) and to clone the protein-coding parts of a gene, which accelerates the engineering of new biological therapies (cDNA cloning, *see* p 38).

RNA takes several different forms (Table 1.1). Although mRNA makes up very little of the total it is the most informative because it tells us which genes are being transcribed. mRNA can be used to make complementary DNA (cDNA, *see* p 37), and DNA copies of all of the mRNA in cells or tissues form a cDNA library. Ribosomal and transfer RNA are rarely prepared deliberately, but the characteristic size of the four types of rRNA can be useful in confirming the presence of RNA in samples

---

Denaturation

Biological molecules have a natural configuration that is necessary for their activity. When this native configuration is disturbed or destroyed, the molecule is said to be *denatured*. For proteins, the configuration is determined during initial folding by the interaction of smaller structural elements such as sheets, coils and helices. For DNA, the principal structural element is its double-stranded nature. Thus, DNA is denatured when it is made single stranded and renatured when the double strand is reformed. RNA is a single strand that folds to form double-stranded regions. RNA is denatured when these regions are made single stranded.

---

prepared for analysis of mRNA, which is very heterogeneous in size.

RNA preparation is more difficult because *ribonucleases* (*RNases*, enzymes that degrade RNA) are extremely stable and can even refold and regain activity after complete denaturation.

To avoid degradation, methods of isolating RNA seek to:

1 inhibit cellular RNases;

2 separate RNA from DNA and proteins (including RNases);

3 keep RNase out by wearing gloves and using bottles, pipettes, etc. that have been treated (e.g. by autoclaving or baking) to destroy RNase.

Detecting and measuring nucleic acids

Fluorescent 'staining' of DNA and RNA

Ethidium bromide (2,7-diamino-10-ethyl-9-phenyl phenanthridinium bromide, EtBr) is a small molecule that inserts (intercalates) between the nucleotides of DNA or RNA and strongly fluoresces under UV illumination. Fluorescence is a phenomenon where a compound is excited by absorbing light at one wavelength and relaxes by emitting light at a different wavelength. In this case, the exciting UV light is literally invisible and a longer-wavelength, visible light is emitted. This forms the basis of a quick, easy and sensitive detection system or 'stain' of nucleic acids. When EtBr binds to DNA or RNA, it is effectively concentrated and its fluorescence increases, so the nucleic acid shows up as a bright band on a dim background of unbound EtBr.

Newer, improved stains are gradually replacing EtBr. For example, a stain called SYBR Green I fluoresces more brightly than EtBr upon binding DNA, is practically non-fluorescent in the absence of DNA, and is specific for double-stranded DNA. Methylene blue also stains DNA, is visible under normal lighting conditions and does not inhibit

Table 1.1 cDNA library. A collection of DNA sequences that are created in the laboratory from mRNA sequences.

RNA name (aliases)	What is it?	How much is there?	How is it prepared?
Total	All the RNA in the cell	~1% of cell mass	Guanidinium lysis, then phenol extraction or CsCl ultracentrifugation
Cytoplasmic	Non-nuclear	Most of the total	Lysis with low detergent concentrations, which keeps nucleus intact; purify RNA from cytoplasm
Messenger (mRNA) (poly A$^+$)	RNA possessing a 'tail' of A nucleotides	*Very* little (3% total)	Prepare total or cytoplasmic RNA, purify poly(A$^+$) by binding ('annealing') to a poly(T) DNA (oligo dT) column, then wash and elute by denaturing the RNA–DNA hybrids
Ribosomal (rRNA)	Structural components of ribosomes	Most of the total RNA	Rarely prepared. Largely the leftover when mRNA is removed from total RNA Four sizes: 28S (4718 bp), 18S (1874 bp), 5.8S (160 bp) and 5S (120 bp)
Transfer (tRNA)	Adapters between mRNA and amino acids	Plentiful	Rarely prepared. About 100 different forms, 75–85 bp in length

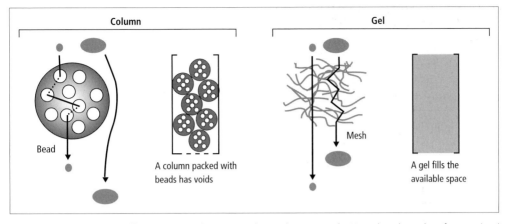

Figure 1.24 Molecules of different sizes can be separated on columns or gels. Note that the order of separation is reversed: larger molecules pass more quickly through the column but more slowly through the gel.

enzymes that act on DNA. These dyes are also said to be less mutagenic than EtBr.

Gels and columns: separation by size

Gels and sizing columns separate molecules in opposite order: small molecules come out of a gel *first* and out of a column *last*. This is because a gel is a mesh that large molecules have a relatively hard time getting through, whereas columns contain beads with small pores that exclude large molecules, but allow in small molecules (Figure 1.24). Since the small molecules can enter the beads, the volume of the column is bigger for them, whereas the excluded large molecules 'see' only the volume between the beads. This is called the *void volume* because it is made up from the voids left between the beads that pack the column. Therefore, larger molecules come out (elute) in a smaller volume (earlier).

The fluid in both columns and gels usually contains a buffer chosen to resist changes in pH. Molecules move through a column in the bulk flow of fluid, driven by gravity or by a pump. In contrast, molecules are driven through a gel by a voltage gradient. DNA and RNA are uniformly negatively charged and naturally adopt a stretched, rod-like configuration. This means that sieving of nucleic acids is a function of their length, unlike proteins that normally fold up compactly and have to be denatured with anionic

detergent to be resolved according to polypeptide chain length.

DNA is negatively charged at neutral pH so it migrates towards the positively charged electrode. The discrete size fragments are usually called 'bands'. Note that the *amount* of DNA in a band, not the size of the DNA in a band, determines the amount of EtBr bound and the resulting fluorescence (Figure 1.25). Confusion on this point is perhaps a consequence of the typical experiment in which a particular DNA is digested and the resulting fragments are analysed by gel electrophoresis. Equal numbers of smaller and larger fragments are generated. However, any particular larger fragment fluoresces brighter than a smaller fragment because it has more base pairs per molecule and comprises more mass. An example of such a digestion is in the right lane of Figure 1.25, labelled 'Size standards'.

Nucleic acids are often detected in the gel stained with EtBr and illuminated by UV light (Figure 1.25). This stain can detect as little as 1ng of DNA in a single band. EtBr is mutagenic and toxic, so solutions and gels must be handled with gloves and disposed of properly. Also, UV light can burn the retina and the skin. Gloves and UV blocking safety glasses are worn when DNA fragments resolved on gels are prepared. EtBr combined with UV light also damages DNA and RNA, so exposure of the sample should be minimized.

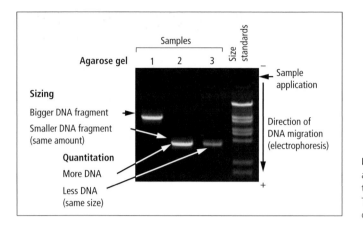

Figure 1.25 Analysis of DNA by agarose gel electrophoresis allows the estimation of size and quantity. The DNA is detected with a fluorescent ethidium bromide 'stain'.

Analysis of RNA by Gel Electrophoresis

Mammalian rRNA produces two prominent bands of lengths 4718 and 1874 bp, called 28S and 18S, respectively (p 17). If these bands are sharp and the 28S band is about twice as bright as the 18S band, then the RNA preparation has probably not suffered significant digestion by RNases. Although the smaller 5.8S (160-bp) and 5S (120-bp) rRNAs are present in equal numbers (they are all subunits of the ribosome), their small size makes them relatively difficult to detect *on gels*.

Really big pieces of DNA, such as even a relatively small piece of a chromosome, cannot be separated by conventional gel electrophoresis. This is probably because the DNA begins to snake through the gel and only small differences are seen in the movements of short versus long snakes. Pulsed field gel electrophoresis (PFGE) was developed to separate large pieces of DNA. The voltage gradient (field) is periodically reorientated so that large pieces of DNA cannot remain orientated 'end-on' and separation by size is possible.

DNA preparation

DNA is prepared so that it can be analysed to gain information about a specific gene, which will answer clinical and research questions or so that multiple copies (clones) can be made. DNA can be prepared in its natural form from chromosomes of eukaryotic organisms and from circular genomes or plasmids of prokaryotes, or synthesized as a complementary strand that matches a mRNA molecule (cDNA).

DNA cloning is the process whereby fragments of DNA can be amplified many times by inserting them into a 'cloning vector', which replicates in bacterial or yeast cells.

Chromosomal DNA: long and stringy

Chromosomal (genomic) DNA is difficult to prepare without shearing (tearing apart) at least some of the DNA. This is hardly surprising when one considers that the DNA contained in one mammalian cell is nearly 2-m long (stretched end to end and deprived of packaging proteins), so the DNA from even a few cells can produce quite a knot. Even the much shorter chromosomal DNA from bacteria (~1 mm) can become a mess quickly and irreversibly.

When large pieces of DNA (>50 000 bp) are needed intact cells can be first embedded in a gel. They are then lysed, protein is removed, and the DNA digested right in the gel (*in situ*). This avoids manipulation that could shear long pieces of DNA. Fortunately, it is rare that very large pieces of DNA need to be analysed intact. The more common, practical problem is that chromosomal DNA is extremely difficult to transfer from one tube to another because it is so stringy (viscous).

Lengthening, shortening and editing DNA

DNA can be lengthened by adding nucleotides using DNA polymerase (p 8), or shortened by removing nucleotides with exonucleases (*see* p 12). In addition it can be cut at specific sites using restriction enzymes, and join back together using DNA ligase (p 32).

Cutting and pasting DNA – restriction enzymes and ligase

Restriction endonucleases are enzymes that cut (digest) DNA at specific sequences (sites).

Editing DNA with enzymes

Molecular biology is founded on the ability to cut DNA at specific places, producing fragments that can be recombined in different ways (recombinant DNA). Restriction endonucleases and ligases are the enzymes that perform these functions.

Restriction enzymes

Restriction endonucleases with over 200 different sequence specificities have been characterized; therefore, many different fragments can be generated. For example, the enzyme *Eco*RI ('echo R one', isolated from **E**scherichia **c**oli) cuts DNA at the sequence GAATTC, whereas *Pst*I (isolated from a different bacterium) cuts at the sequence CTGCAG (Figure 1.26).

Commonly used restriction enzymes typically recognize symmetrical DNA sequences (Figure 1.27). This symmetry is a consequence of the fact that these enzymes are homodimers, composed of two identical protein subunits.

Note the importance of the $5' \rightarrow 3'$ orientation as a convention for writing DNA sequences (Figure 1.28). *Eco*RI, which cuts the sequence 5'-GAATTC, would not cut the same sequence of nucleotides in the opposite orientation (3'-GAATTC). As it happens, the restriction enzyme *Afl*II would cut this sequence (5'-CTTAAG).

> ### Restriction and Modification – Bacterial Defence
>
> Restriction enzymes are purified from a variety of bacteria, which use them for defence against viruses called bacteriophages (literally 'bacteria eaters'). Bacteriophage DNA is said to be *restricted* (cut) by a bacterial strain when it cannot infect that strain of bacterium. Bacteria avoid cutting their own genomic DNA by *modifying* it, particularly through methylation, rather than forbidding these DNA sequences. Modification systems vary amongst bacterial strains. Mammalian DNA can usually be cut by restriction enzymes *in vitro* because eukaryotic methylation patterns differ from those of bacteria (prokaryotes). (In eukaryotes, DNA methylation is involved with gene expression and compaction.) Ironically, restriction enzymes allow molecular biologists to generate recombinant DNA plasmids, which they introduce into and grow in bacteria. In the laboratory, bacterial strains mutant in one or more of the *restriction–modification* (R-M) system enzymes are used as hosts to reduce incompatibility problems. All commonly used restriction enzymes are type II, which recognize symmetrical DNA sequences, cut symmetrically, and leave 3'-hydroxyl and 5'-phosphate ends. Type II restriction enzymes are dimers of single polypeptides, which are easier to mass produce than are multisubunit enzymes. The rarely used type I and III restriction enzymes contain multiple subunits. They recognize specific sequences but do not cut exactly or completely.

The examples given above are all 6-bp recognition sites. The six-base cutters are used most often because they tend to cut DNA into fragments that are small enough to handle yet big enough to be useful. The average fragment length is a function of the size of the recognition sequence and the approximately random distribution of A/T/G/C in DNA (ignoring for now the fact that the mammalian genome is AT-rich and CG-poor). With four bases to choose from, a given sequence of six base pairs occurs once every approximately 4000 bases ($4^6 = 4096$) by chance. In contrast, an 8-bp cutter like *Not*I is more useful for mapping larger pieces of DNA such as mammalian genomes, because it produces only one-sixteenth as many DNA fragments (of an average 64 000 bp). Over 2000 restriction enzymes have been isolated to date, with around 200 different sequence specificities, which means that there are usually several

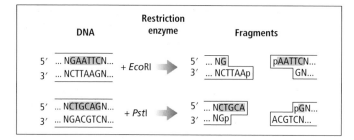

Figure 1.26 Different restriction enzymes cut different sequences. 'N' means any DNA base and only the new terminal phosphate (p) is shown.

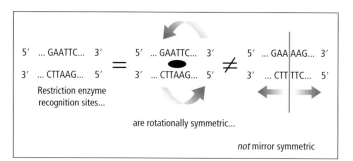

Figure 1.27 Nearly all commonly used restriction enzymes cut rotationally symmetrical sequences. Recognition sequences are often said to be palindromes, as in the phrase 'Madam, I'm Adam' (in which the comma/apostrophe is rotationally symmetrical).

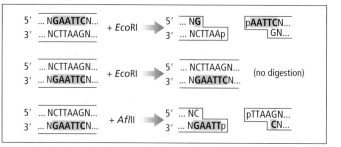

Figure 1.28 Orientation is important because 5'-GAATTC is not the same as 3'-GAATTC.

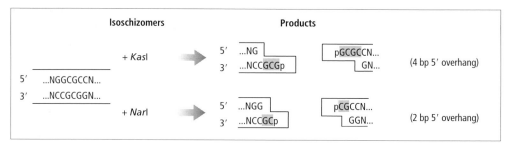

Figure 1.29 Isoschizomers are different restriction enzymes that recognize the same sequence but may cut in different ways.

enzymes that recognize a given sequence. When different restriction enzymes recognize the same sequence, they are called *isoschizomers*. They do not always cut at the same place in the sequence (Figure 1.29).

The frequency of certain restriction enzyme sites is actually much lower than expected. As noted above, mammalian genomes are A- and T-rich, which reduces the frequency of restriction sites containing G or C. Even so, the frequency of the CG dinucleotide is fivefold lower than would be expected based on G and C content alone. Consequently, restriction enzyme sites containing CG are relatively rare in mammalian genomes. Furthermore, these CG sites are often methylated, which is a modification that blocks cutting by many restriction enzymes. Surprisingly, the genome is not homogeneous in this respect: stretches of several hundred to thousand bp, called CG dinucleotide 'islands', are found in which the CG dinucleotide occurs at nearly the expected frequency. Often, these islands are found 5' of genes, an early observation that has since led to the identification and cloning of several genes based solely on their position downstream (3') of CG islands (*see* Chapter 2).

Ligases

DNA ligase takes two ends and connects the phosphate backbone. Three types of ends can be ligated: blunt, 'sticky' and single-strand nicks.

Sticky ligations are more efficient because the compatible ends stick together (anneal), albeit weakly (Figure 1.30). On the other hand, blunt-end ligations are particularly useful because of the ability to recombine any DNA fragments, without a need for compatible ends (Figure 1.30). DNA ligase also heals 'nicks' in DNA, where *one* of the two phosphate backbone chains is broken.

Several practical considerations enter into ligating DNA fragments (Figure 1.31). Blunt-cut vectors can close without any DNA being inserted. This unwanted product of self-ligation can be reduced by dephosphorylating the vector, in which case ligation depends on the phosphate groups at the ends of the insert. Vectors with different 'sticky' ends cannot close on themselves because the overhanging ends are not compatible (they do not anneal to one another). Sticky-end ligation with different ends permits 'directional cloning', since the insert can only 'go in' one way.

Amplifying DNA – polymerase chain reaction (PCR)

Polymerase chain reaction (PCR) is used to make many copies of ('amplify') fragments of DNA. This simple but incredibly powerful technique has revolutionized molecular biology and many applications are already mainstays of clinical and forensic medicine. You can easily generate many copies of a single target DNA, such as a viral gene. With some modification, it can also be used to calculate the amount of target DNAs. The recipe is simple, just add the ingredients (template, oligo primers, nucleotides, buffer, polymerase) and bake (and cool, bake again and cool . . . , Figure 1.32).

Polymerase chain reaction amplifies the segment of DNA between the oligonucleotide primers, which are usually 15–25 bp long and designed to match specific sequences (5' and 3') flanking the segment to be amplified. Therefore, it is *usually* necessary to know these flanking sequences (although methods have been developed allowing PCR amplification of segments when the sequence of

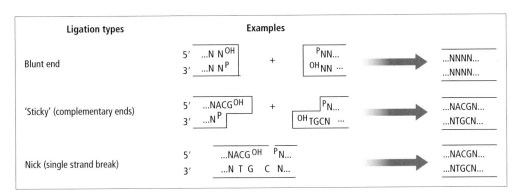

Figure 1.30 DNA ligase catalyses the formation of a bond juxtaposed between 5'-phosphate (P) and 3'-hydroxyl (OH) groups on the phosphate 'backbone' of DNA.

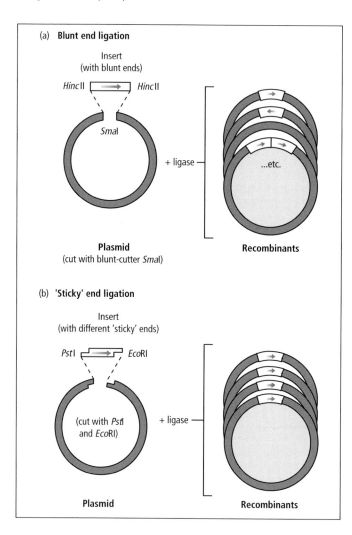

(a) Blunt end ligation

Insert
(with blunt ends)

*Hinc*II   *Hinc*II

*Sma*I

+ ligase

...etc.

Plasmid
(cut with blunt-cutter *Sma*I)

Recombinants

(b) 'Sticky' end ligation

Insert
(with different 'sticky' ends)

*Pst*I   *Eco*RI

(cut with *Pst*I
and *Eco*RI)

+ ligase

Plasmid

Recombinants

Figure 1.31 DNA fragments can be recombined with ligase. (a) Blunt end ligations can combine fragments from different restriction enzyme digestions but the products are heterogeneous. (b) 'Sticky' end ligations combine only fragments with matching restriction enzyme digestion – producing overhangs but the products are uniform.

only one end is known). DNA polymerase extends the primers after they anneal to the template, creating a duplicate, complementary strand.

PCR was first described using bacterial DNA polymerase and the reaction tubes were moved manually to different temperatures. Fresh enzyme was added for each thermal cycle because the enzyme was destroyed at the temperatures required to melt the DNA. These flaws in an otherwise beautiful procedure spurred the production of *heat-stable enzymes*, the first of which to be widely used was *Taq* DNA polymerase (from *Thermus aquaticus*), a bacterium found in hot springs), and

automated thermal cycling instruments. Many additional thermal stable DNA polymerases, RNA polymerases and DNA ligases, as well as sophisticated instruments, are now available.

Accelerating PCR analysis (faster!)

The rate-limiting step in PCR is often the detection and analysis of the amplified product. Several methods have been devised to quickly determine the presence of the product by using thermal cyclers that detect fluorescence during cycling.

1 *Fluorogenic DNA stains.* Product accumulation can be monitored using stains that fluoresce upon

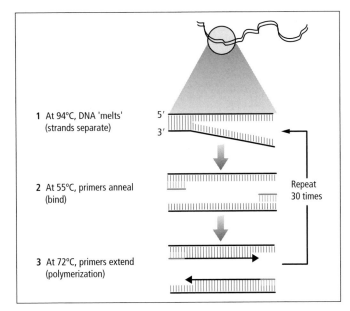

Figure 1.32 'Some like it hot'. One thermal cycle in the PCR is shown. Steps 1–3 double the amount of template flanked by the primers. Repeated 30 times, they yield a million-fold amplification in about 1 h.

Figure 1.33 The phenomenon called fluorescence resonance energy transfer (FRET) underlies many new analyses. (a) Fluorescence occurs when light energy at a certain frequency excites a compound, called a fluor, which then relaxes by emitting light at a second frequency. Here, incident blue light excites and green light is emitted. A second fluor is not excited by blue light. (b) When different fluors are close enough (approximately 5 nm, or two times the width of a double-stranded DNA helix), an excited donor fluor can transfer energy without light emission directly to a second acceptor fluor. The second fluor emits light at a different frequency, here red. (c) A special acceptor called a quencher efficiently absorbs the fluorescence of the first fluor but does not itself fluoresce.

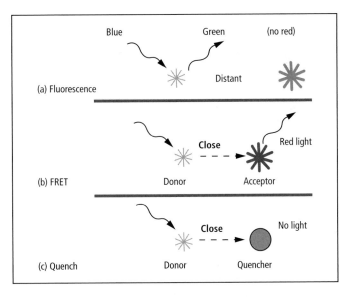

binding to double-stranded DNA and do not inhibit DNA polymerization, for example, SYBR Green I.

2 *FRET* is a very sensitive measure of the distance between two different molecules (Figure 1.33). This phenomenon has been applied to measuring specific PCR products (Figure 1.34). In contrast to the use of fluorogenic stain, specific FRET probes permit the detection of multiple templates

amplified simultaneously in one sample, a process known as multiplexing.

Two FRET adaptations are widely used for continuous 'real-time' measurement. One known as Molecular Beacons uses a probe that forms a hairpin loop, juxtaposing the donor and quencher (Figure 1.34(a)). At annealing temperatures, the 5–7 nucleotide 'arms' can form the stem, or the

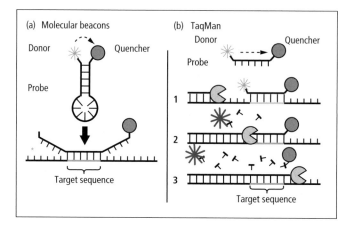

Figure 1.34 Fluorogenic assays accelerate PCR analysis. (a) With molecular beacons, a donor fluor is fixed to the 5′ end of an oligonucleotide and a quencher is fixed to the 3′ end. The complementary ends form a short stem in a hairpin loop structure. The sequence in the middle of the probe anneals to the target sequence, disrupting the loop and separating the quencher from the donor. (b) With TaqMan, the donor fluor and quencher are fixed to the opposite ends of the probe oligonucleotide, which anneals to the target sequence. During PCR, the exonuclease activity of Taq clears the path ahead of the polymerase activity by degrading the probe oligo, separating the fluor from the quencher.

loop of 10–40 nucleotides can bind to the target sequence, resulting in fluorescence. A second assay called TaqMan ('Tack man') is named after the old video game character, Pac-Man, that eats everything in its path (Figure 1.34(b)). The assay depends on the 3′–5′ exonuclease activity of Taq, which normally clears a path ahead of the 5′–3′ polymerase activity. Single-stranded probes annealed to the template are degraded by Taq, freeing the fluorescent reporter from the quencher.

Isothermal nucleic acid amplification – some like it cooler . . .

Future amplification systems may not use thermal cycling but instead hold a steady temperature,

Rolling Circle Amplification

Rolling circle amplification (RCA) is modelled on the replication of circular DNAs such as the genomes of bacteria and some viruses. A primer oligonucleotide, usually tethered to a location by a variety of means, is annealed to a circular template and extended by polymerase. Unlike the amplifications described above, which occur in solution, RCA has the unique attribute of being easily localized. This is useful for *in situ* analyses, such as histology, and gene 'chips' (*see* p. 44).

that is, isothermal. Room-temperature or 'warm' amplification/detection systems may have particular application in clinical testing, where time is critical and thoroughly tested reagent kits can be prepared for specific assays. For example, the amplification of pathogen-specific DNA or RNA may allow the rapid identification of infections or monitoring of a patient's response to treatment. The 'rolling circle' isothermal amplification system is being used now as a detection system in pathology and to amplify whole genomes in genetic analysis.

Making DNA from RNA – RNA polymerase and reverse transcriptase

In the beginning, the word was that genetic information could go in only one direction, from DNA to RNA to protein. The dogma was shaken when it was found that viruses with an RNA genome (retroviruses) replicate through a DNA intermediate, so information was moving from RNA to DNA (and then back to RNA). The descriptive name *reverse transcription* was given to this activity, and the responsible enzymes are called reverse transcriptases (RT, Figure 1.11).

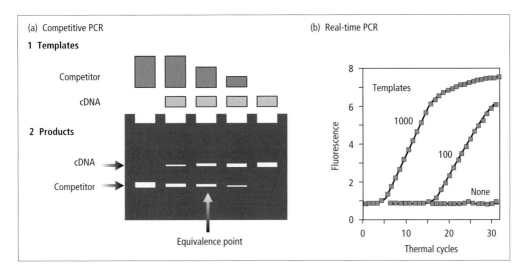

Figure 1.35 Templates can be quantified by PCR. (a) In competitive PCR, a constant amount of cDNA and a known amount of competitor template is added to each reaction. Control reactions at each end contain only competitor template or cDNA. The products are analysed on an agarose gel. The equivalence point, where the intensities of the competitor and cDNA bands are equal, is a measure of the specific RNA from which the cDNA was generated. (b) Real-time PCR is performed in special thermocyclers that can read fluorescence. With more templates in the initial mixture, the product accumulation is detectable earlier.

Complementary DNA

cDNA is DNA that 'complements', or matches, mRNA. cDNA is synthesized as the opposite or complementary strand of mRNA. To make cDNA, RNA is first prepared and then reverse transcribed. All mRNAs possess a poly(A) tail (a string of A ribonucleotides that is added to the 3′ end of mRNA after transcription), whereas rRNA and tRNA, which make up the bulk of total or cytoplasmic RNA preparations, do not. Oligo dT (a string of T *deoxy*ribonucleotides) is often used to prime the first strand synthesis by RT, because it anneals specifically to the poly(A) tail and can thereby selectively prime cDNA synthesis from mRNA. The second strand is more difficult to synthesize and several methods have been developed (Figure 1.36).

DNA Cloning

DNA cloning is the production of multiple identical copies of a DNA fragment in the laboratory.

Cloning Vector

A cloning vector is a DNA molecule from a virus, plasmid, cosmid, phage, bacteria or yeast into which another DNA fragment of appropriate size can be inserted, and then introduced into host cells where the DNA can be reproduced in large quantities.

Plasmids are circular, double-stranded DNA molecules that replicates within bacteria independently of the chromosomal DNA.

Cosmids are very large plasmids, which contain *cos* sites (cohesive sequences) that allow them to be packaged into bacteriophages.

A bacteriophage is a virus that infects bacteria, sometimes referred to as a phage.

Amplifying DNA made from RNA – reverse transcription-PCR

When coupled with PCR amplification, RT can provide the only means of measuring very small amounts of RNA, much less than is necessary for other techniques such as a northern blot in which RNA separated by gel electrophoresis is transferred to a membrane for detection

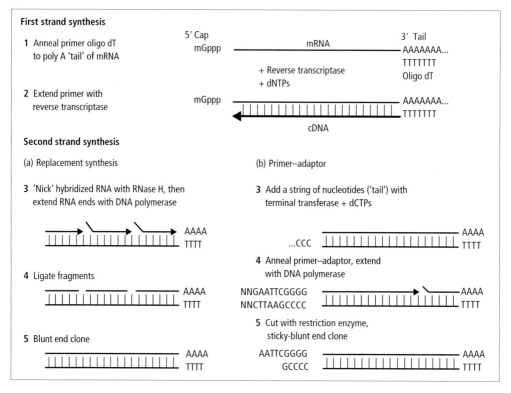

Figure 1.36 cDNA can be cloned by two different methods. Synthesis of the first cDNA strand is primed by a short strand of thymine nucleotides (oligo dT) which bind to the poly(A) tail of mRNA. Second strand synthesis is more difficult and two of the many different protocols are shown. (a) Replacement synthesis is simple, but the extreme 5′ end is lost because there is no primer further upstream to replace the RNA. Ligation proceeds despite this RNA end and the cap. (b) The primer–adaptor method is more complicated but it can clone the 5′ end. For this method, the oligo dT primer in the first strand synthesis often also contains a restriction site, which permits directional cloning into expression vectors.

(*see* p 41). The RNA is reverse transcribed by RT using oligo dT or six-base oligonucleotides with random sequence ('random oligos') that anneal all over the RNA. These act as primers that are extended to produce a cDNA strand, which is then amplified by PCR.

Reverse transcriptase-PCR (RT-PCR) is therefore used to amplify very small amounts of mRNA so that they are easier to detect or analyse. The key elements of RT-PCR are:

1 Make cDNA from RNA with RT and oligo dT primers.

2 PCR amplify cDNA with gene-specific primers.

3 Analyse PCR products.

RT-PCR is excellent for determining whether a gene is transcribed and can be used to measure large differences in mRNA levels, but it is poor at reliably measuring smaller differences (10-fold and less). This is because slight differences in the efficiency of PCR amplification produce large differences in product, independent of the original amount of template. For example, the difference between an efficiency of 80 and 85% yields a difference of more than sixfold after 30 cycles ($1.6^{30} = 1.3 \times 10^6$ versus $1.7^{30} = 8.2 \times 10^6$). A modification, called *competitive PCR*, controls for differences in amplification efficiency by including in every sample different, known amounts of a distinguishable template (Figure 1.35). The point in the titration at which the cDNA and the added competitor template produce an equal amplification is then taken as a measure of the original cDNA amount.

Copying DNA – cDNA cloning

A clone is a population of genetically identical organisms, cells or molecules that derive from the replication of a single progenitor.

DNA can be cloned by inserting the DNA into a cloning vector, or in cell free systems using polymerase chain reaction (p 32).

Plasmid DNA: small and circular

Plasmids are small, circular DNAs that are independently replicating in bacteria because they have their own origin of replication (*ori*). Bacteria have always exchanged useful genes using plasmids; molecular biologists have been using plasmids only in the last couple of decades. Plasmids are quite easy to isolate from bacteria, manipulate *in vitro* and reintroduce into bacteria.

Plasmids are often used as *cloning vectors* because the DNA to be cloned can be inserted into the

plasmid and then 'grown up' along with the rest of the plasmid DNA, resulting in thousands, even millions of copies of the DNA segment of interest. Using recombinant DNA techniques, plasmids have been improved for use as cloning vectors in the following ways (Figure 1.37):

- Addition of restriction enzyme sites (*see* p 32) that allow the plasmid DNA to be cut at particular sites (e.g. the polylinker) to permit incorporation of the DNA fragment of interest.
- Addition of genes that allow simpler screening and selection procedures (*see* p 45) to find successful recombinants.
- Removal of non essential DNA to make the plasmid smaller and deletion of restriction enzyme sites (e.g. the *Eco*RI site formerly at position 1), which makes the plasmid easier to manipulate.
- Substitution of a mutant origin of replication (*ori*) that allows *relaxed copy number* control, meaning that the plasmid continues to replicate after the bacterium has stopped. Although not desirable for the bacterium or the symbiotic plasmid, this is great for producing a much higher yield of DNA for the molecular biologist.

Plasmid DNA can be transferred into mammalian cells through a process called *transfection* (p 45). The transfected plasmid is usually lost after a few rounds of cell division but it can occasionally become incorporated into genomic DNA, producing a stable transfectant. There are also

Yeast and Bacterial Artificial Chromosomes– YACs + BACs

Yeast artificial chromosomes – DNA segments, containing up to 2 million base pairs and having a centromere and telomere can be introduced into the yeast *Saccharomyces cerevisiae* allowing the cloning and isolation of much larger DNA segments than is possible using bacterial cloning.

Bacterial artificial chromosomes are propagated as stable inserts of about 150 000 in *E coli.*

Plasmids Are Circular

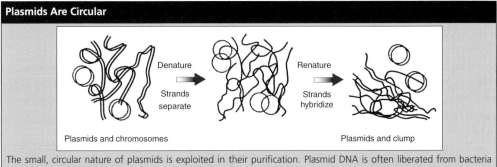

The small, circular nature of plasmids is exploited in their purification. Plasmid DNA is often liberated from bacteria under denaturing conditions, which cause the DNA strands to separate. Upon renaturation, the complex bacterial chromosomal DNA strands cannot readily find their matching strand and instead form short, weak double-stranded regions. In contrast, the circular plasmid DNA strands are able to rapidly reanneal following denaturation, making them easy to separate by centrifugation.

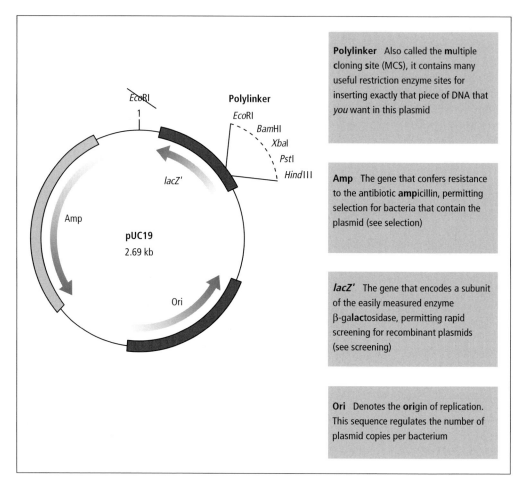

Polylinker Also called the multiple cloning site (MCS), it contains many useful restriction enzyme sites for inserting exactly that piece of DNA that *you* want in this plasmid

Amp The gene that confers resistance to the antibiotic **amp**icillin, permitting selection for bacteria that contain the plasmid (see selection)

lacZ' The gene that encodes a subunit of the easily measured enzyme β-galactosidase, permitting rapid screening for recombinant plasmids (see screening)

Ori Denotes the **ori**gin of replication. This sequence regulates the number of plasmid copies per bacterium

Figure 1.37 Plasmids are the workhorses of molecular biology. For example, the plasmid pUC19 (for plasmid Universal Cloning 19) is a second-generation, relatively simple, cloning vector of 2686 bp (2.7 kb) that was constructed from parts of earlier plasmids using recombinant DNA technology. Plasmids are often named with a p (for plasmid) followed by identifying letters (sometimes the initials of the molecular geneticist who designed the plasmid) and the edition number. Numbering of the base pairs starts at the top marked '1' and proceeds clockwise. During the construction of pUC19 an *Eco*RI restriction enzyme site that was originally at this position was deleted, as indicated by the line through the name, to maintain a unique *Eco*RI site in the polylinker.

plasmids that include pieces of animal viruses such as SV40 (simian virus 40) or retroviruses that enable their autonomous replication in mammalian cells. Yeast and mammals also have natural circular, independently replicating, extrachromosomal DNAs (e.g. mitochondrial DNA), but they are larger, do not possess screening or selection functions or multiple cloning sites (sites with a short DNA sequence in a cloning vector that contain several restriction enzyme sites), do not

replicate in bacteria, and so they lack many of the attributes of a good cloning vector.

Here are several reasons why cDNA cloning is popular and powerful:

• cDNA is shorter than genomic DNA which contains all the gene's exons, introns and untranslated regions. Some relatively small proteins are encoded by incredibly large genes, possessing long introns and UTRs. Dihydrofolate reductase (DHFR), for example, has a protein-coding region of

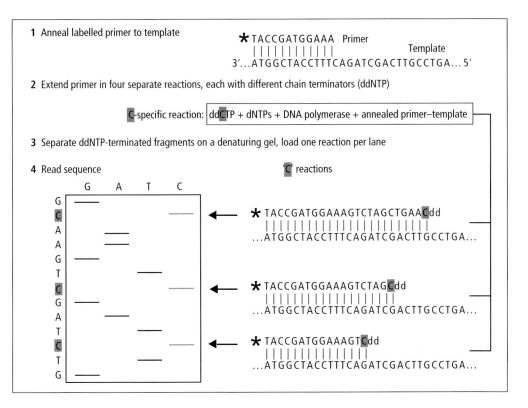

1 Anneal labelled primer to template

★ TACCGATGGAAA Primer

| | | | | | | | | | | | Template

3′...ATGGCTACCTTTCAGATCGACTTGCCTGA...5′

2 Extend primer in four separate reactions, each with different chain terminators (ddNTP)

C-specific reaction: ddCTP + dNTPs + DNA polymerase + annealed primer–template

3 Separate ddNTP-terminated fragments on a denaturing gel, load one reaction per lane

4 Read sequence   'C' reactions

G   A   T   C

G
C
A
A
G
T
C
G
A
T
C
T
G

★ TACCGATGGAAAGTCTAGCTGAACdd
| | | | | | | | | | | | | | | | | | | | |
...ATGGCTACCTTTCAGATCGACTTGCCTGA...

★ TACCGATGGAAAGTCTAGCdd
| | | | | | | | | | | | | | | | | |
...ATGGCTACCTTTCAGATCGACTTGCCTGA...

★ TACCGATGGAAAGTCdd
| | | | | | | | | | | | | |
...ATGGCTACCTTTCAGATCGACTTGCCTGA...

Figure 1.38 DNA sequencing using dideoxy chain terminators is also known as Sanger sequencing. Note that only a fraction of each reaction is terminated by the addition of dideoxynucleotide (ddNTP) at each corresponding nucleotide position. Otherwise, no sequence would be obtained beyond the first nucleotide. Fluorescent nucleotides are often used instead of a radioactive primer.

approximately 600 bp distributed over a gene that is 31 500 bp.

• cDNA contains the most important parts. The exons are usually the more interesting part, at least initially, because their sequence affords what is often the first glimpse into what the protein looks like.

• cDNA can be made from RNA that is enriched for the mRNA of interest by using particularly high-expressing cells or by treating cells to induce the mRNA, whereas for the genomic DNA only two copies are present in each and every (somatic) cell. cDNA cloned using the mRNA from specific cells or tissues will contain coding information for proteins that are expressed. The clones form a cDNA library.

When gene sequencing was extremely expensive, cDNA was the easiest way to focus analysis on the most information-rich part of the genome. Researchers produced large collections of cDNA clones called expressed sequence tags (EST) libraries), which were valuable for finding genes, for analysing gene structure, and for establishing landmarks in the genome.

cDNA also helps in cloning genes and producing recombinant proteins because the introns are eliminated, often greatly reducing the size of the DNA to be cloned and expressed. Using cDNA, one can clone and analyse the protein-coding part of a gene and then proceed directly to producing the protein in large quantities as a recombinant protein. Also, recombinant proteins (p 42) encoded by cDNA can be produced in bacteria, which do not have introns and do not have the splicing mechanisms to remove introns.

DNA Sequencing

DNA is sequenced to determine the order of the nucleotides.

DNA and RNA analyses

DNA sequencing

There are two ways to sequence DNA, the hard way using noxious chemicals or the modern way using enzymes and inexpensive kits. (Then there is the easiest way, using a commercial service.) These methods involve analysing the DNA of interest in four different nucleotide-specific reactions that remain incomplete, each reaction yielding a heterogeneous population of molecules that terminate at one particular nucleotide. The enzymatic method of sequencing, also called *Sanger* sequencing after its developer, uses

*di*deoxynucleotides (ddNTPs). Unlike normal deoxynucleotides (dNTPs), ddNTBs cannot be extended by DNA polymerase. These populations of molecules are then resolved on a denaturing polyacrylamide gel, one lane per nucleotide-specific reaction (Figure 1.38).

In chemical sequencing, also called *Maxam–Gilbert* sequencing after the developers, the sequence is obtained from the DNA itself, instead of an enzymatic copy. The DNA to be sequenced is labelled at one end and then treated with chemicals that specifically destroy one or two of the nucleotides (either purines or pyrimidines or only one nucleotide). The reactions are not allowed to go to completion, otherwise only the shortest product would remain and no sequence 'ladder' would be obtained.

A modification of the DNA sequencing technique uses a thermostable polymerase, as used in PCR, and repeatedly anneals, extends and melts.

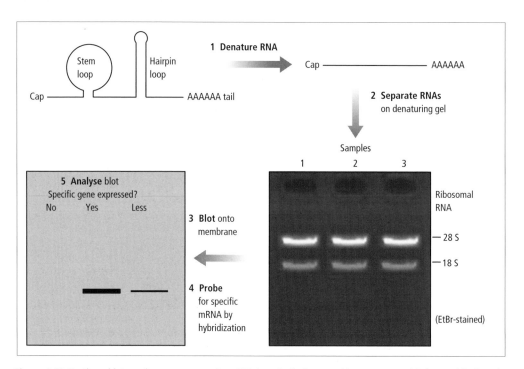

Figure 1.39 Northern blots analyse gene expression. RNA is typically denatured by treatment with formamide then size separated on a denaturing agarose/formaldehyde gel. Along with quantifying the amount of mRNA, mRNA size can be estimated by comparison to the rRNA or to size standards run in a separate well. Using less stringent probe hybridization conditions could also test the expression of similar genes (homologues).

Although no chain reaction is established in this procedure because the product does not act as template in the next round, it can provide a sequence from very little DNA template. The elevated extension temperature also reduces interference from secondary structures in the template and simplifies sequencing double-stranded DNA.

Gene chips – parallel analysis

RT-PCR (p 47) and Northern blotting (p 42) detect and quantify specific individual RNA molecules.

Northern blot

Northern blots are used to identify, quantify and determine the size of mRNA species. In a Northern analysis (Figure 1.39), RNA molecules of different sizes are resolved on a denaturing formaldehyde gel, the gel is blotted and the blot is hybridized

with a labelled probe (Figure 1.40). The denaturing gel unfolds the RNA so that separation is based on length alone and not on secondary structure such as hairpin loops. The formaldehyde in the gel reacts with the denatured nucleotides and prevents their refolding. The formaldehyde is soaked out of the gel and away from the RNA before blotting.

However, modern technology often requires large-scale measurement of how the genome is being transcribed to provide the 'big picture', analysing how thousands of genes are being transcribed even when it was not known what you are expecting to find. Gene chips follow a trend towards miniaturization, which allows fast analysis of many genes that are being expressed in small biological samples.

mRNAs are usually converted to more stable cDNAs (*see* p 37), which are quantified by hybridization to thousands of complementary gene sequences spotted onto glass slides

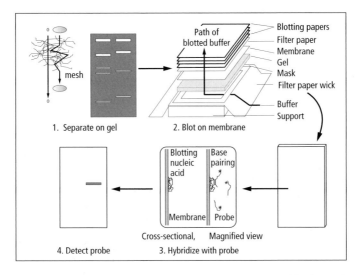

Figure 1.40 Blotting and hybridization. 1. Molecules of different sizes can be separated by driving them through a gel mesh by a voltage gradient. Negatively charged RNA or DNA moves towards the positive electrode, and smaller molecules move more quickly. 2. Blotting carries nucleic acids out of gels and onto membranes. The stack of filter papers, gel, membrane and blotting paper is held out of the buffer bath by the support. The blotting papers absorb buffer and wicking action (absorption) pulls the buffer up through the gel, carrying the nucleic acids along, and then through the membrane, to which the nucleic acid binds. The mask ensures that the buffer goes through the gel rather than around it. 3. The blot is hybridized with a sequence-specific probe. Hybridization is the formation of base pairs between nucleic acids. The blot is hybridized with a labelled (easily detectable) piece of DNA or RNA called the probe. 4. The method of detection depends on the type of label on the probe. Typically, the probe is radioactively labelled and detected on photographic film (autoradiography).

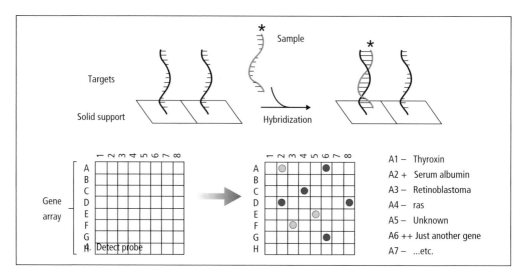

Figure 1.41 Gene 'chips' can identify transcripts. The sample nucleic acid (DNA or RNA) is often marked with a fluorescent dye. The target DNA is bound to solid support, in a highly organized spatial order.

Blotting Nucleic Acids and Proteins

In a Southern blot, DNA is separated by movement through a non-denaturing gel, then denatured with sodium hydroxide and blotted. The blot is then probed with either labelled DNA or RNA. The gel may also be a denaturing urea/polyacrylamide gel, in which case denaturation prior to transfer is not necessary. The Southern blot is named after its originator, Dr Edwin Southern.

In a Northern blot, RNA is separated by movement through an agarose gel containing a denaturing agent (formamide/formaldehyde) and blotted. The blot is then probed with labelled DNA or RNA. The Northern blot was named whimsically after the Southern blot.

In a Western blot, proteins are separated by movement through a gel containing a denaturing detergent (sodium dodecyl sulphate (SDS)/polyacrylamide gel), and then blotted and detected with antibodies. To complete the naming, DNA-binding proteins are detected in a South-western blot and RNA-binding proteins are detected in a North-western blot. In these assays, proteins are separated and then probed with nucleic acids. The future directions in blotting techniques seem clear.

glass slides. Researchers then attach fluorescent labels to DNA or RNA samples they are studying. The labelled probes bind to the DNA strands on the slides, and the slides are scanned to measure how much of the specific nucleic acid of interest is present in the sample. The genes arrayed on the chip may be chosen for particular profiles. For example, DNA from a tumour may be characterized using an array of genes that include tumour suppressors and oncogenes.

Instead of probing many different genes in one sample, it is also possible to probe many different samples with one gene. Gene chips may be made with copies of a patient's gene, which is fixed on a slide and then probed with oncogenes or other disease-related genes. For example, chips have been used to detect mutations in the cystic fibrosis gene (*CFTR*), a breast cancer gene (*BRCA1*) and the oncogene p53. The classification of cancers such as melanoma has benefited from the ability to assess the global gene expression simultaneously throughout the genome.

(Figure 1.41). The strategy, in other words, is to look everywhere and figure out what you're looking for later.

The process uses a robot to precisely apply tiny droplets, each containing a specific DNA, onto

Serial analysis of gene expression – one tag at a time

As attractive as 'gene chips' are, the future of gene expression studies may actually use a technology that is less immediately tractable. The serial analysis of gene expression (SAGE) technique does not directly measure the expression level of a gene, but quantifies a 'tag', which represents the mRNA transcript of the gene. SAGE relies on the fact that a short (10–24) nucleotide sequence can uniquely identify a given mRNA transcript. These sequences act as a 'tag'. If the tags are adjacent to restriction sites they can be cut out of the transcript, linked together, cloned, sequenced and analysed efficiently by machine. The data produced is a list of tags, which can be quantified according to their frequency giving a digital readout of cellular gene expression.

Beadarray – light at the end . . .

A new type of microarray (BeadArray technology™, Illumina) uses optical fibres that hold latex beads coated with short DNA probes at one end. The beads will bind complementary nucleotide sequences when exposed to DNA in a sample, and the beads have a fluorophore and a quencher that are close to each other when no DNA from the sample is bound. When DNA binds the quencher is displaced and the fluorophore regains its fluorescence. A bundle containing up to 50 000 individual fibres, each holding an individual bead, is exposed to a DNA sample and light is then passed down the optical fibre from the other end, exciting the fluorescent

label on the beads to which complementary DNA has bound.

Transposition – natural recombination

A *transposon* is a piece of DNA, often flanked by specific repeat sequences, that can be efficiently excised from or integrated into a second DNA molecule. Transposition is a highly efficient means of generating recombinant DNA molecules. Several enzyme systems employed by organisms ranging from bacteria to mammals are involved in the reversible insertion of a piece of foreign DNA into the genomic DNA of a host.

Nature has produced the variety of life without recourse to a laboratory. Molecular biologists have only recently begun to exploit transposition to generate recombinant DNA. The ease with which DNA pieces can be moved around threatens to take some of the art and craft out of molecular biology (Figure 1.42).

Some transposons are called retrotransposons because of their similarity to RNA viruses (retroviruses). Integrated retroviruses may account for about 1% of the human genome. These are called human endogenous retroviruses (HERVs), although chimpanzees and gorillas have largely the same endogenous retroviruses, suggesting they are very old. Human disease has been attributed to transposition. One HERV on chromosome 7 is suspected of

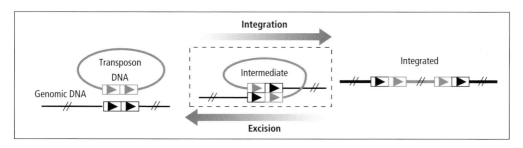

Figure 1.42 Transposition is precise and reversible. During integration, similar or identical sequences within the transposon DNA and genomic DNA align. Both DNAs are cut within the repeat and rejoined with the other DNA. The integrated DNA that results can still be identified by the presence of flanking, direct repeat sequences. The transposon can also be excised from genomic DNA. In bacteria, these reversible reactions require only three enzymes: bacteriophage-encoded integrase (Int) and excisionase (Xis) and a bacterial protein called integration host factor (IHF).

causing testicular and other cancers. A different retroviral insertion causes a form of congenital muscular dystrophy by interfering with the expression of a secreted protein. The potential transfer of endogenous retroviruses between species is also a concern that might limit the therapeutic transplantation to humans of tissues from different animals (xenotransplantation).

Putting genes back into cells – transfection and transformation

Two different names are given to the process of putting genes back into cells. Bacterial cells are said to be *transformed* because in a classic experiment non-pathogenic bacteria were made pathogenic by addition of the 'transforming principle', that is DNA. Mammalian cells are *transfected* because the transfer of genes is similar to viral infection. Both cell types spontaneously pick up DNA, but the efficiency is very low. Numerous transfection techniques have been developed to increase the efficiency of uptake:

- Calcium phosphate precipitation – DNA forms aggregates that precipitate and are endocytosed by the cells.
- DEAE-dextran – this cationic gel and DNA form large aggregates, which are endocytosed.
- Cationic liposomes – coat the (anionic) DNA in lipid so that it passes more readily through the cell membrane.
- 'Biolistics' – DNA is coated onto gold particles that are shot into the cells or tissues.
- Electroporation – creates transient DNA-permeable holes in the cell membrane by a high-voltage shock.
- Infection ('transduction') – genes are 'packaged' into infectious viral particles.

Transfection of mammalian cells often results in only a small fraction of the cells receiving DNA into their nucleus. This DNA is typically not replicated and rapidly diluted or lost from the nucleus upon cell division. A few cells become stable transfectants by incorporating the transfected DNA into their chromosomes. Many experiments are designed to find out what you want to know *before* the DNA is lost from the cell. These are called *tran-*

Transduction Is Virus-Mediated Gene Transfer
Genetic material can be transferred from one bacterium to another by a bacteriophage (*see* Box titled "Analysis of RNA by Gel Electrophoresis", p 29). Viruses that naturally infect human cells, including both DNA viruses (such as adenovirus) and RNA viruses (such as retroviruses) can be modified and used as vectors to efficiently transfer genes into target cells.

sient transfections (or simply transients) because they last only a few days.

Finding cells that have acquired designer genes – selection and screening

With the low efficiency of transformation and transfection, there is a need to identify the cells that have taken up DNA by either *screening* or *selecting* positive clones. An example of selection is when bacteria are transformed with a plasmid containing a gene that confers antibiotic resistance (*see* Figure 1.38). The few cells that take up the plasmid and express the gene will be able to grow in medium containing the antibiotic, such as ampicillin, while the other cells will not (Figure 1.43). Similarly, stable mammalian cells transfected with a gene for resistance to a toxin can be selected in a toxin-containing medium. G418 or hygromycin B are examples of these toxins.

Alternatively, a plasmid that contains a gene encoding a protein that can be detected in transformed or transfected cells can be used. This is *screening* for expression. A commonly used gene encodes the enzyme β-galactosidase (β-gal), whose activity can be assayed with substrates that change colour. For example, the β-gal-catalysed conversion of a colourless compound called Xgal (the real name is very long) to a blue precipitate allows the identification of transformed bacteria or transfected animal cells (Figure 1.44).

Many experiments use a combination of selection and screening to assess whether the DNA of interest had been taken up into the cell.

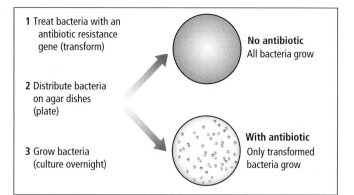

Figure 1.43 Antibiotics select for transformed bacteria. Bacteria that pick up the DNA containing the ampicillin resistance gene are able to grow on agar containing ampicillin (antibiotic resistance). The transforming DNA usually includes additional genes that are not so easily selected.

Figure 1.44 Blue/white screening for bacteria containing normal and recombinant *lacZc* marker genes. The *lacZc* gene encodes a critical portion of the enzyme b-galactosidase (b-gal). When cultured in the presence of Xgal (a chromogenic substrate of b-gal) and an inducer of b-gal expression, bacteria that synthesize b-gal can be found because they turn blue. Screening is usually combined with simultaneous selection for antibiotic resistance.

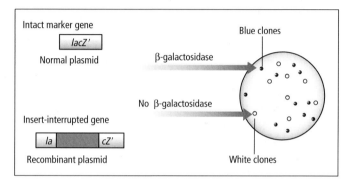

Recombinant proteins

Recombinant DNA technology allows the production of large quantities of pure proteins for clinical practice and research. The proteins produced by these techniques are termed recombinant even when they are identical to the natural proteins. Many recombinant human proteins are used in clinical practice (*see* Chapter 3).

Once the gene for a particular protein has been cloned, it is inserted into plasmid under the regulation of a strong promoter. Such a construct is called an *expression vector* because it is designed to express large amounts of protein. Different promoter sequences are used depending upon whether the protein is to be made in bacterial, yeast or mammalian cells. The expression vector encoding the recombinant protein is then transfected into the genome of microorganisms or cultured mammalian cells, which then produce the protein.

Making mutants

Site-directed mutagenesis is used to prepare specific mutants (variants) of a known gene. At last, here is an art, in the form of biotechnology, that improves on nature. Natural mutants are generated *randomly*, through mistakes in DNA synthesis or repair, and most are deleterious. The rare beneficial mutation could still be lost unless it happens to be very beneficial, such as when the alternative is extinction. Even with accelerated mutagenesis and screening/selection *in vitro*, this is too slow, far too slow, for your biotechnologist 'on

Oligonucleotides

An oligonucleotide is a short sequence of DNA, usually containing less than 25 nucleotides. Oligonucleotides are often prepared synthetically for use as PCR primers or as probes to see if the complementary sequence is present in a DNA sample.

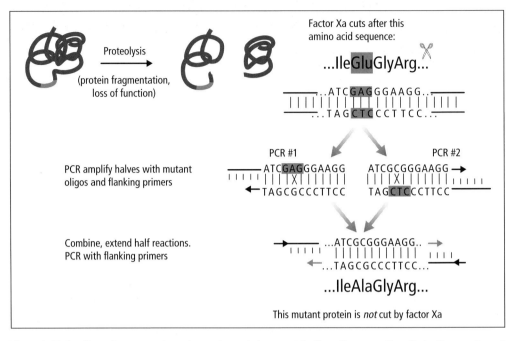

Figure 1.45 Site-directed mutagenesis can be used to redesign a protein. Here, the recognition site for the complement enzyme factor Xa, is mutated. The resulting protein is not cleaved and might be more stable *in vivo*.

the go'. Synthetic oligonucleotides are the answer for quick (and, with PCR, easy) designer genes.

Site-directed mutagenesis is a technique that introduces base pair changes at specific locations in target DNA. In general, changes are limited to one or two base pairs with the intention of changing a codon encoding an amino acid, a restriction site, or sometimes a regulatory element in a gene. A synthetic DNA fragment is used as a template to change one or more base pairs (*see* Figure 1.45), and the reprogrammed DNA codes for a different amino acid sequence. The importance of a particular amino acid to the structure or function of a particular protein can then be studied, and proteins with altered function can be synthesized.

Chapter 2

Understanding genetics

Genes encode all of the cell's RNAs and proteins, which constitute the structural components and signalling molecules of an organism or act as enzymes to direct the formation of these components, such as lipids and carbohydrates. Here we will review how genes are inherited, how they are identified as discrete entities in the genome, how they can change (mutate), and how these changes can influence health. Finding mutations and determining how they affect health and disease are key goals of current biomedical research. Correcting or compensating for mutations is the goal of gene therapy.

Historical primer – traits, genes, DNA

Gregor Mendel, an Austrian monk, determined the basic laws of inheritance by observing how seven traits of garden peas were passed down though several generations. He concluded that each trait is independent of the others and transmitted by two particles, one inherited from each parent. We call these particles *alleles*, which are versions of a single gene. For example, flower colour is a trait encoded by a gene with several alleles; one allele produces white flowers and another produces purple flowers. Alleles for these traits are passed unchanged to the next generation independent of the alleles of other genes. This means that no 'blended' alleles encoding intermediate shades of colour are generated.

Mendel's insight was enabled by two simplifications. First, he followed discrete traits with unambiguous expression patterns encoded by a single gene. For example, purple flower colour is dominant over white flower colour, which we would call a recessive trait. Second, he followed traits that happen to be entirely independent because they are encoded by genes that are not physically connected, as we now know. Although Mendel formulated these laws around 1860, their publication in an obscure journal delayed their widespread acceptance for many years.

Gene, Alleles and Traits

A *gene* is a DNA sequence that encodes a trait and, typically, an RNA. An *allele* is one sequence version of a gene. Many different alleles may exist in a population.

Mendel's rules apply to human traits and heritable diseases, a fact that was first noted by Garrod in 1900. Genes were given a physical form soon thereafter, when Sutton postulated that genes are carried on previously identified structures called chromosomes ('coloured bodies'), so named because they can be stained and observed by light microscopy. The physical linkage of some genes on the same chromosome explained the co-inheritance of these genes and added new laws. These laws of inheritance were elucidated in peas and fruit flies by Bateson, Punnett and Morgan (1910).

Genes are made of DNA, first shown by Avery and colleagues (1940). The DNA sequences are linked end to end, forming enormously long molecules that are packaged with specialized proteins into chromosomes. Genomic DNA is composed of two complementary, anti-parallel strands, which assumes a double helix shape. Watson and Crick determined this structure (1950), which immediately suggested mechanisms for replication by unzipping the helix and using one strand as a template to copy the other complementary strand. McClintock (1950) revolutionized genetics by showing that the genome is dynamic and that genes and whole chromosomal regions can move (*see* Transposition). Increasing complexity should not obscure the fundamental observation that all living things employ essentially identical genetic materials and mechanisms of inheritance.

Some Genes Hardly Change

Essential cellular functions are often performed by gene products that change very slowly through evolution. For example, negatively charged DNA is neutralized by the basic chromatin protein histone 2A. This protein is identical in *garden peas* and *humans* at 93 out of 118 amino acids.

Transmitting genes – Mechanisms of inheritance

Mendel's laws summarize the results of a few key physical events that underlie patterns of inheritance. All the cells in the body except the germ cells (eggs in females or sperm in males) are called *somatic* cells. Human somatic cells have 23 pairs of chromosomes. Males and females possess equivalently 22 of these chromosomes, numbered 1–22 and called the autosomes. For the twenty third pair, called the sex chromosomes, females possess two X chromosomes while males possess one X and one very small Y chromosome. The X–Y sex chromosomes are very dissimilar and can pair only on their short arms (Xp : Yp). Each chromosome has a specialized region called a centromere ('central thing')

that is responsible for the movement of the chromosome into daughter cells (Chapter 1, p 35). The ends of chromosomes, called telomeres ('distant things'), consist of large numbers of short repeat sequences that are maintained independent of replication by the enzyme telomerase.

Chromosome Ends are Special

Telomeres in humans consist of as many as 2000 repeats of the sequence TTAGGG. They keep the ends of chromosomes from accidentally becoming attached to each other. Telomeres gradually shorten with DNA replication and below a critical length cell division stops. The enzyme that maintains telomeres, *telomerase*, is a reverse transcriptase that adds telomere repeat sequences to the end of DNA strands. By lengthening the strand before replication, cells with telomerase activity are able to compensate for telomere shortening during DNA replication. Telomerase activity is found in embryonic stem cells and in the vast majority of tumour cells, but is almost absent from somatic cells.

Somatic cells are *diploid*, meaning that each chromosome is present in two copies (one pair). One member of each pair is derived from the father and the other from the mother. As cells divide, the genome is perpetuated through the process of mitosis. Mitosis is divided into several stages corresponding to events that are visible in the light microscope (*see* Chapter 1).

Duplicating and Distributing Genes at Cell Division

Mitosis copies the genome and distributes *both* alleles to diploid daughter (somatic) cells. *Meiosis* separates chromosome pairs and distributes *single* alleles to haploid germ cells.

Meiosis – forming germ cells

In developing germ cells, the diploid germ cell progenitors replicate their genomes once and divide twice (meiotic division), resulting in half as many chromosomes per (haploid) germ cell. Thus, a human germ cell (an egg or a sperm) has one member of each chromosome pair, that is, 23 *unpaired* chromosomes. An egg and a sperm unite to form a fertilized ovum or zygote, which develops into a new human being with a unique combination of chromosomes.

First meiotic division – replicate, recombine and divide

Before the first meiotic division, the germ cell progenitors replicate their DNA just as they would if they were undergoing mitosis. This produces doubled chromosomes composed of two identical *sister chromatids*. At this point, the cell contains double the normal amount of DNA, a condition called *tetraploid* (Figure 2.1). No further DNA replication occurs during meiosis. During the next process, called prophase, chromosomes condense and become visible, revealing the two identical sister chromatids held together at the centromere. The sex chromosomes X and Y pair along a short homologous 'pseudoautosomal' region.

In a process unique to meiosis, the homologous chromosomes closely align and form synapses during late prophase. The paired chromosomes exchange segments at this stage through the process of crossing over and *recombination* . Then the pairs of sister chromatids segregate into the daughter cells. After the first meiotic division, each daughter cell contains one pair of sister chromatids of each chromosome. Although they contain the normal amount of DNA, these are not normal diploid cells because the chromatids are identical, except for any changes resulting from recombination.

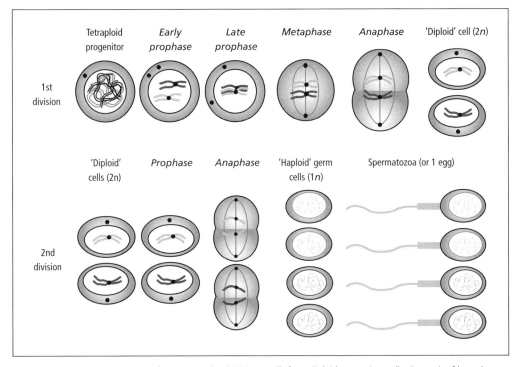

Figure 2.1 Meiosis is the process of generating haploid germ cells from diploid progenitor cells. One pair of homologous chromosomes is shown. DNA is replicated before meiosis begins. In late prophase, the homologous sister chromatids pair and engage in crossing over, generating recombinants. Instead of containing 1 copy of each allele, the diploid '2n' cells shown here are duplicated haploids, containing 2 copies of only 1 allele.

Second meiotic division – divide and segregate

During the second meiotic division, the paired chromosome strands divide at the centromere. Each daughter germ cell receives 23 *single* chromosomes, one member of each original chromosome pair (Figure 2.1). In males, all four haploid cells develop into sperm. In females, however, only one of the four haploid cells develops into an egg. The other three haploid cells, called polar bodies, are very small cells; this conserves the progenitor cell cytoplasm for a single large egg. The first meiotic division occurs in human females before their birth and the second meiotic division is completed during ovulation, when the egg matures. In males, meiosis does not begin until adolescence and continues thereafter throughout adult life.

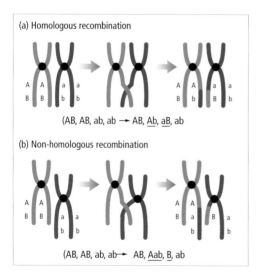

(a) Homologous recombination

(AB, AB, ab, ab → AB, <u>Ab</u>, <u>aB</u>, ab)

(b) Non-homologous recombination

(AB, AB, ab, ab → AB, <u>Aab</u>, <u>B</u>, ab)

Figure 2.2 Recombination occurs where chromatids cross over during prophase in meiosis, generating recombinant chromatids (underlined). (a) Homologous recombination occurs when paired chromatids cross over. Here, two loci are shown with two alleles at each locus (*A* or *a* and *B* or *b*). After crossing over occurs, there are two chromatids of the parental haplotype (*AB* and *ab*) and two recombinant haplotypes (*Ab* and *aB*). (b) Non-homologous recombination (unequal crossing over) occurs when different regions of the chromosomes pair. The result is two parental chromatids (*AB* and *ab*), one chromatid with a gene duplication (*Aab*) and one with a gene deletion (*B*).

Genes on different chromosomes have a 50% chance of being inherited together because chromosomes segregate into germ cells independently. Genes on the same chromosome *may* be inherited together, depending on how close they are. The further apart the genes, the greater the chance that they will be separated by recombination (Figure 2.2). Overall, the chance of recombination is roughly 1% per million base pairs (Mbp). Since chromosomes average 100 Mbp in length, genes even on the same chromosome often segregate practically independently. However, recombination does not occur randomly. For example, recombination is particularly common within certain highly repetitive DNA sequences, raising the possibility that such sequences may be involved in promoting recombination (*see* below).

Homo/Hetero/Hemizygotes

An individual with identical alleles of a given gene is *homozygous* at that genetic locus. A *heterozygote* has two different alleles. A *hemizygote* has only one allele (e.g. many genes on the X and Y chromosomes in males).

Recombination is the generation of DNA sequences from combinations of old sequences, which occurs when pairs of condensed chromosomes (chromatids) 'cross over' while they are juxtaposed at synapses during prophase (Figure 2.2). Homologous recombination occurs between *similar* DNA sequences. Non-homologous (unequal crossing over) occurs between less similar parts of the chromosomes and can result in the deletion of DNA from one chromatid and its duplication on the other. This creates variations in length and may cause the reciprocal loss and duplication of a gene. Multigene families (*see* below) are thought to have arisen through this process. Non-homologous recombination is less common than homologous. Chromosome ends are protected from recombination by telomeric repeat sequences.

Dominant and Recessive Alleles

A trait encoded by a *dominant* allele is expressed regardless of the second allele. Dominant alleles are represented by uppercase letters (*A*) and recessive with lower case letters (*a*). A trait encoded by a *recessive* allele is expressed only in homozygotes, in which both alleles are the same.

Genes that are close together on a chromosome tend to be inherited together rather than independently. Such genes are *linked*. The tendency of genes to be coinherited forms the basis of *linkage analysis*, which maps genes relative to measurable traits (*see* below).

Genotype encodes Phenotype

A *genotype* is the complement of genes possessed by an individual. A *phenotype* describes the physical characteristic resulting from expression of the genotype.

Mendel's laws

Mendel summarized his findings in two laws:
1 *Segregation: The two alleles for each gene segregate into different germ cells* (sperm or eggs).
2 *Independence: Genes controlling different traits assort independently.*

These conclusions stood in contrast to the views of Mendel's contemporaries, who wrongly believed that parental traits blended inextricably in the progeny (Figure 2.3). Mendel's laws fit our understanding of many gene behaviours.

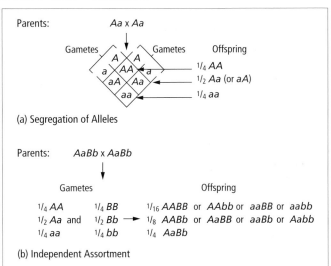

Parents: *Aa* x *Aa*

Gametes   Gametes   Offspring

    $^1/_4$ *AA*
    $^1/_2$ *Aa* (or *aA*)
    $^1/_4$ *aa*

(a) Segregation of Alleles

Parents: *AaBb* x *AaBb*

Gametes   Offspring

$^1/_4$ *AA* $^1/_4$ *BB* $^1/_{16}$ *AABB* or *AAbb* or *aaBB* or *aabb*
$^1/_2$ *Aa* and $^1/_2$ *Bb* → $^1/_8$ *AABb* or *AaBB* or *aaBb* or *Aabb*
$^1/_4$ *aa* $^1/_4$ *bb* $^1/_4$ *AaBb*

(b) Independent Assortment

Figure 2.3 Chromosome distribution into developing germ cells underlie Mendel's simple laws of heredity.

Figure 2.4 The Punnett Square helps visualize independent segregation of the alleles and the frequency of the offspring. (a) Heterozygous parents with one dominant and one recessive allele of a given gene, symbolized as *Aa*, generate equal numbers of gametes containing each allele, *A* or *a*. Heterozygous parents (*Aa* × *Aa*) produce offspring in these ratios: 25% *AA*, 50% heterozygotes (*Aa* or *aA*) and 25% *aa*. (b) A larger square is necessary to trace two alleles, so it is easier to calculate the odds of particular genotypes using allele frequencies.

(a)   <u>*Aa*</u>

	Gametes	*A*	*a*
Aa	*A*	*AA*	*Aa*
	a	*aA*	*aa*

(b)   <u>*AaBb*</u>

	Gametes	*AB*	*Ab*	*aB*	*ab*
AaBb	*AB*	*AABB*	*AABb*	*AaBB*	*AaBb*
	Ab	*AABb*	*AAbb*	*AaBb*	*Aabb*
	aB	*aABB*	*aABb*	*aaBB*	*aaBb*
	ab	*aABb*	*aAbb*	*aaBb*	*aabb*

Parents heterozygous at one locus can produce heterozygous or homozygous offspring. This process can be visualized with a Punnett Square (Figure 2.4(a)). Parents heterozygous at two different genes (*Aa* and *Bb*) give rise to progeny with several different genotypes (Figure 2.4(b)). It is easy to calculate the offspring genotypes using the *allele frequency* (Box "Genotype encodes Phenotype).

Allele Frequencies are Stable

The ratios of alleles in a population, their *allele frequencies*, change very slowly through generations. Only the combinations of alleles change quickly. For example, the progeny of *AaBb* x *AaBb* will tend to possess each allele in the same frequency as the parents, 50% each allele: *A*, *a*, *B* and *b*. This is true despite the fact that only 25% of the progeny would have the same genotype (*AaBb*) as the parents. Double homozygotes would be the rarest (*AABB* or *aabb*, each 1/16 = 6%). The stability of allele frequencies is fundamental to evolution and disease genetics.

Patterns of inheritance

Most traits are encoded by genes within the nuclear genome and are inherited according to the patterns first described by Mendel. Non-Mendelian patterns are due to influences of the cytoplasm, which is inherited almost exclusively from the mother. These cytoplasmic effects are mediated either by proteins influencing nuclear genes or by genes within the mitochondria.

Mendelian (traditional) inheritance

Four different patterns of inheritance depend on whether the nuclear gene is dominant or recessive

and whether it is carried on the X chromosome or an autosome. Y-linked diseases are nearly unknown in humans. Typical Mendelian patterns of inheritance can be demonstrated in families in which a trait can be tracked through several generations (Figure 2.5; Pedigree). The most clinically relevant traits are caused by changes in genes that predispose to certain diseases, often through disruptions in a metabolic or signalling pathway.

1 Autosomal recessive – affects people of either sex whose parents are usually both asymptomatic carriers. The risk of having an affected child is increased if the parents are related because the two inherited alleles are more likely to be identical. A single copy of an autosomal recessive allele is carried usually without effect (no phenotype). If both parents are carriers (*Aa* × *Aa*), each child has a 25% chance of being affected, a 50% chance of being a carrier, and a 25% chance of not inheriting either copy of the mutant gene (*see* Figure 2.4). If only one parent is a carrier (*Aa* × *AA*), each child has a 50% chance of being a carrier but essentially no risk of being affected.

2 Autosomal dominant – affects people of either sex; the mutation is either inherited from one parent or arises *de novo*. Even a single copy of an *autosomal dominant* allele causes or influences the phenotype. Each child of an affected parent has a 50% chance of being affected.

3 X-linked recessive – almost always affects males. Each son of a carrier mother has a 50% chance of being affected while each daughter of a female carrier has a 50% chance of being a carrier, like her mother. There is no father to son transmission. In females, usually both X chromosomes must be

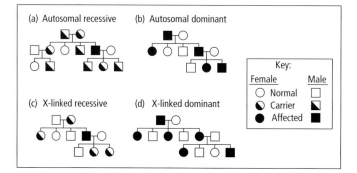

(a) Autosomal recessive (b) Autosomal dominant

(c) X-linked recessive (d) X-linked dominant

Key:

Female | Male
○ Normal | □
◑ Carrier | ◪
● Affected | ■

Figure 2.5 Pedigree charts demonstrate representative patterns of Mendelian gene inheritance. For recessive alleles, homozygotes are affected and heterozygotes are asymptomatic carriers. For dominant alleles, there are no carriers because heterozygotes are affected. A *proband* is the first affected member that brings a family to the notice of a physician.

mutant to produce a phenotype. Heterozygous daughters may show some mild disease characteristics because of non-random inactivation of the X chromosome (*see* below).

4 X-linked dominant (XLD) – affects daughters more often, but usually less severely, than sons. Daughters are less affected because they also receive a second X chromosome from the unaffected parent. Sons are usually more severely affected, and some XLD alleles are lethal, because their sole X chromosome is the disease-carrying chromosome. In the next generation, sons of an affected father are unaffected because their X chromosome is from their mother. Daughters of an affected father are always affected because one of their X chromosomes is inherited from their father. Each child of an affected mother has a 50% chance of being affected.

Disease alleles

The frequency of disease-causing alleles is usually very low. These alleles are generated by genetic change (*mutation*) and are slowly removed as a consequence of their deleterious effects, a balance called *mutation-selection*. Some disorders are caused by many different alleles; other disorders are usually caused by a single, *common* allele. For example, nearly every third case of the blood coagulation disorder haemophilia B is caused by a distinct mutation of the clotting factor IX. Nearly three-quarters of these alleles arose in independent mutations. The most common allele, thought to have derived from a single common ancestor, accounts for only 5% of the families in the United Kingdom. In contrast, over two-thirds of cases of the respiratory and digestive system disorder cystic fibrosis (p 57) are caused by the same mutation in an ion channel protein (del F508, shorthand for 'deletion of a phenylalanine amino acid at position 508 in the protein'). About 5% of the US population carry the del F508 allele. Why did this mutant allele become so common? Perhaps because when it is paired with a non-mutant ('*wild type*') allele (i.e. a heterozygote), it may increase resistance to bronchial asthma and reduce diarrhoea in response to pathogens. There are many other, less frequent mutant alleles that can cause cystic fibrosis, but each only accounts for an average of 1 in 100 European cases of the disease.

Trinucleotide repeat disorder

These disorders, caused by many repeats of a three nucleotide pattern, exhibit unique inheritance patterns. The hallmark of trinucleotide repeat disorders is *genetic anticipation*, which is the tendency through generations for the disease to increase in severity and develop earlier. Both increased severity and earlier onset correlate with the increasing numbers of repeated trinucleotides. Recall that three nucleotides comprise a codon, which encodes an amino acid; several of these diseases are characterized by aberrant proteins with repeated amino acids. *See* Chapter 3 for details about selected trinucleotide repeat disorders.

> **Genetic Anticipation**
>
> Genetic anticipation is a pattern of disease worsening over generations. In trinucleotide repeat disorders, disease severity and earlier onset correlate with increasing numbers of repeats.

Fourteen trinucleotide repeat disorders that affect humans have been documented and more probably await identification and characterization. Eight of these fourteen are caused by repeated CAG, which encodes glutamine, and are collectively known as the polyglutamine diseases. These repeats occur in different proteins and even different chromosomes, distinguishing the disorders. In Huntington disease (p 122), for example, the repeat occurs in 'huntingtin' (i instead of o), a protein encoded by a gene on chromosome 4 that was identified in a study of unrelated patients. Between 9 and 30 CAG repeats in huntingtin are normal; disease is evident in individuals with 39 or more copies. In the disease Dentatorubropallidoluysian Atrophy (DRPLA), the repeat occurs in atrophin-1, a protein encoded on chromosome 12. Asymptomatic individuals have between 6 and 35 CAG repeats; disease has been found in individuals with 49–88 copies. Polyglutamine diseases are characterized by gradual nerve cell degeneration, often culminating in nerve cell death. By adulthood, muscle weakness and reduced coordination are usually evident, often together with more troubling symptoms. Other symptoms vary according to the organ or tissue most affected.

The disease Spinocerebellar Ataxia Type 12 (SCA12) is also caused by CAG repeats. However, it is not a polyglutamine disease because these repeats do not occur within the protein-coding region of the gene. Instead, the repeats are found in the 5' ('upstream') *untranslated region* (UTR) of PP2A, a brain-specific regulatory subunit of a protein phosphatase. Repeats in UTRs may influence RNA stability, perhaps by altering structures such as hairpin loops that can stabilize RNA. Note that such changes in RNA stability could also contribute to the effects observed in protein-coding region changes because the longer- or shorter-lived mRNA could yield more or less protein.

Other trinucleotide repeat disorders are caused by different repeats. Several of these are also non-protein coding. Myotonic dystrophy (p 122), for example, results from a CTG repeat in the 3' ('downstream') UTR of the *DMPK* gene on the long arm of chromosome 19 (19q13.3). Fragile X Syndrome (FRAXA) results from expansions of a CGG repeat in 5' UTR of the fragile X mental retardation gene (*FMR1*) on the X chromosome. The repeats correlate with increased methylation and silencing of *FMR1* transcription. FRAXA is the most common form of inherited mental retardation after Down syndrome. FRAXA patients display specific cognitive defects. Unique sequences or single nucleotide variants are used to diagnose FRAXA patients (e.g. DXS548 or rs4949; *see* STS and SNP).

Repeats expand due to replication slippage (new strand mispairing and shifting on the template), mistakes in DNA repair, and through recombination (e.g. unequal sister-chromatid exchange). Repeat expansion can also occur in somatic cells, so mitotic as well as meiotic mechanisms can operate. Repeats that can form hairpin loops, including CAG and CGG repeats, may expand particularly rapidly. Also, the propensity of DNA to 'slip' during replication is proportional to the length and homogeneity of the repeat. In some places in the genome, repeats can be innocuous and even useful as markers for gene mapping (*see* microsatellite).

Non-Mendelian inheritance

Imprinting

Most genes behave the same whether they are inherited from the mother or the father. However, a few genes are active only when they are inherited from the mother and others only when they are inherited from the father. In these cases, the genes received from the other parent are silenced during the development of the egg or sperm (gametes), a phenomenon known as *genetic imprinting*. Studies suggest that 10–25% of the mouse genome is imprinted; the fraction of the human genome that is imprinted is unknown.

Imprinted genes are clustered in the genome. The cluster is silenced by the enzymatic addition of a methyl group to the cytosine of specific CpG dinucleotides within the cluster, thereby reducing transcription of the nearby genes. Methylation is a general mechanism of gene regulation performed by a large family of methylases (Figure 2.6). Methylation is a dynamic and genome-wide process.

Upon fertilization, imprinted genes remain methylated despite a genome-wide process of demethylation and remethylation that occurs around implantation. Imprinting is 'erased' early in germ cell development and then re-established about the time of birth. This means that genes are active or imprinted depending solely upon whether they came from the mother or father and independent of whether they came from a grandmother or grandfather.

Developmental problems and disease can result when the active gene is mutant or when the normally imprinted gene is not inactivated. Similarly, as a result of an error, cells may receive all or part of a pair of chromosomes from a single parent (*see* Uniparental disomy). For imprinted genes, that means that the cell receives either two imprinted copies or two active copies, resulting in over- or under-expression. Research has shown that maternal genetic imprinting errors can occur when egg follicles from mice are matured in a culture dish. Such errors may contribute to the abnormal

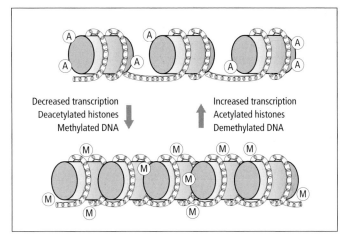

Figure 2.6 Methylation of DNA and acetylation of histones regulate gene expression. Methylated CpG dinucleotides (circled 'M') are associated with reduced gene transcription and compacted DNA. Imprinted genes are heavily methylated. In contrast, acetylated histones (circled 'A') are associated with actively transcribed genes. Acetyl groups are added by histone deacetylases (HDACs) and removed by histone acetyl transferases (HATs).

Decreased transcription
Deacetylated histones
Methylated DNA

Increased transcription
Acetylated histones
Demethylated DNA

development observed in some cloned animals (*see* below). Cancers have been associated with failure to imprint genes; especially genes that produce growth factors (*see* section on Cancer). Selected disorders of imprinting are discussed in Chapter 3.

Aneuploidy

Aneuploidy is a chromosome number different from the normal ($n = 23$). Aneuploidy usually results from a failure of homologous chromosomes to separate during mitosis or meiosis (nondisjunction). The most common changes are one more ($2n + 1$, *trisomy*) or less ($2n - 1$, *monosomy*). The complete absence of one chromosome pair is *nullisomy* ($2n - 2$) while the presence of two homologous chromosomes in a germ cell is *disomy* ($n + 1$).

Trisomy

The most common viable human aneuploidy is trisomy of chromosome 21, resulting in Down syndrome (Chapter 3). Frequency of trisomies increases with maternal age and, less dramatically, paternal age. The reason for the prevalence of the maternal age effect is not established but may be due to the long delay between the first meiotic division, which occurs before birth, and the second meiotic division, which begins in some eggs at the onset of each menstrual cycle.

Uniparental disomy

Uniparental disomy is when two copies of a gene are inherited from one parent and none from the other. The incidence is unknown because it is not always detected. An estimated one in 500 cases of cystic fibrosis is due to uniparental disomy, which is detected when only one parent is a carrier of the common mutation del F508. Uniparental disomy is detected more often when it occurs within a region that is genetically imprinted because these regions behave dramatically differently depending on which parent contributed them.

The most frequent cause of uniparental disomy is an unequal recombination between the chromosomes. Translocation and nondisjunction during the first meiotic division can also cause chromosome imbalance, yielding some gametes with two copies and other gametes with no copies of particular chromosomes. The two chromosome sequences could be identical, a condition called *isodisomy* resulting from the duplication of 1 chromosome, or different, a condition called *heterodisomy* resulting from inheriting both replicated chromosomes. In each case, the chromosomes appear structurally normal by standard chromosome analysis under the light microscope.

Mutations that disturb imprinting of chromosome 15 have been shown to underlie the congenital disorders Prader-Willi Syndrome (PWS) and Angelman Syndrome (AS). Imprinting errors on chromosome 11 underlie Beckwith Wiedemann syndrome. These are discussed in Chapter 3. Uniparental disomy may cause additional, currently mysterious syndromes. Clinicians can suspect uniparental disomy and genomic imprinting when a patient or pedigree or appearance is atypical. For example, a child with cystic fibrosis due to maternal uniparental disomy also has marked short stature, possibly due to missing genes on the paternal chromosome 7.

Mitochondrial

Mitochondria are the site of the respiratory system that oxidizes sugars to generate ATP, the source of energy for cellular metabolism. Mitochondria contain their own DNA (mtDNA, ~17 kbp), which encodes 13 subunits of the respiratory complexes. The remaining subunits are encoded by the nuclear genomic DNA (gDNA), which also encodes transporters of metabolic products as well as factors essential for mtDNA transcription, translation and replication.

Genetic errors in mitochondrial functions contribute to many diseases, including cardiomyopathies, deafness, blindness and Alzheimer disease (Chapter 3). Defects often are revealed in cells with high energy demands and many mitochondria, such as cardiac muscle. Defects encoded by nuclear gDNA are inherited as Mendelian traits. Defects encoded by mtDNA can display a maternal inheritance pattern. The egg contributes much more cytoplasm than the sperm to the fertilized egg. Consequently, the fertilized egg receives nearly all its mitochondria from the approximately 1700 present in the egg. This is the basis of maternal inheritance pattern for mitochondrial defects caused by mtDNA mutations. Specifically, a female carrying a mutation in her mtDNA can pass the mutation onto both sons and daughters, while a male carrying a mutation in his mtDNA cannot pass the mutation.

Mitochondria are Maternally Inherited

You could've inherited your father's Y's but you certainly have your mother's mitochondria.

Contributing to the inheritance pattern is the fact that mutant mitochondria can survive as long as the cell has a sufficient number of capable mitochondria. However, a cost of inefficient energy production is the generation of excess reactive oxygen intermediates, predisposing to cell death and the development of diseases. Mitochondria are also randomly distributed to daughter cells, instead of evenly distributed as are nuclear genes, raising the possibility that daughter cells may receive insufficient numbers. Mitochondrial defects have been treated post fertilization by microinjecting healthy mitochondria into the fertilized egg (ooplasmic transplantation). This has resulted in healthy babies who possess mitochondria from both their mother and the mitochondria donor. Alternatively, the nucleus may be transplanted into a donor egg from which the original nucleus has been removed.

Maternal inheritance of mtDNA allowed researchers to trace human lineage. By comparing mtDNA from 147 people from all continents and estimating the time it would take to generate the diversity they observed, they concluded that the most recent common ancestor is an African woman living about 200 000 years ago. Subsequent estimates ranged between 50 000 and 500 000 years ago.

Genes, loci and alleles – broader definitions

The complexity of genetic organization makes accurate description difficult and the nomenclature is often imprecise. A gene was originally defined as a unit of heredity, encoding a trait. With the advent of molecular tools, 'gene' is used synonymously with any length of DNA encoding an RNA and usu-

---

Genes, Loci, and Regions

A *gene* is a segment of DNA that contributes to phenotype by encoding, or controlling the expression of, a transcript. A *locus* is a point in the genome, mapped to a particular location by a marker. A *chromosome region* is larger than a locus, encompassing several genes or markers.

---

ally a protein, regardless of whether a trait is known to be associated.

This expanded definition of gene includes regulatory DNA sequences that control RNA transcription but are not themselves transcribed into RNA. The more general term *locus*, meaning a point on a line, refers to a physical location of a gene, but remember that genes are not always found in one consistent order on the chromosome. DNA moves and mutates, and is duplicated and deleted, producing chromosomal variation in the human population. Accurate description is challenging and recognition of the nomeclature's limitations improves understanding.

Gene symbols – unique names

Genes have been named for many different reasons. Names were often based on the first identified function, which might not be the major function, and genes identified in non-human organisms were sometimes named whimsically based on phenotype. Even a single activity can have multiple names. For example, peptidase proteinase and protease all describe enzymes that hydrolyze peptide bonds. Informal naming has led to a proliferation of names, with single genes having multiple names and a homologous gene in different species having completely unrelated names.

To help bring order to the naming process, investigators agreed to certain rules. Naming guidelines from the Human Gene Nomenclature Committee were first published in 1979 and have been updated under HUGO. Each gene symbol should:

1 be short, descriptive and unique;

2 contain only upper case Latin letters and Arabic numerals (no punctuation);

3 start with a letter and not end in 'G' (if it stands for 'gene');

4 not contain species reference (e.g. 'H' for human).

All approved human gene symbols and their more descriptive names can be found in *Genew*, the Human Gene Nomenclature Database. For example, the human gene encoding member 10b of the Tumour Necrosis Factor Receptor 'SuperFamily' is abbreviated *TNFRSF10B* (gene names are usually italicized). This single gene product previously had many names, including Fas-like protein precursor, TNF-related apoptosis-inducing ligand (TRAIL) receptor 2, death receptor 5 (DR5), p53-regulated DNA damage-inducible cell death receptor (killer), and many more. As of early 2005, there are over 20 000 approved gene symbols, leaving only an estimated few thousand before all the genes identified by the Human Genome Project have been named.

There are three exceptions to the 'no punctuation' rule, for the immunologically important HLA (Human Leukocyte Antigen), immunoglobulin and T cell receptor gene symbols. These symbols were assigned by World Health Organization (WHO) and 'ImMunoGeneTics' (IMGT) committees and adopted by the human genome nomenclature committee.

Finding Genes – Mutants, Markers and Maps

Genetic discoveries are now influencing decisions in clinical care and physicians are key collaborators in the multidisciplinary teams that are finding disease genes. As a consequence, it is increasingly important that all physicians understand how these discoveries are made. A deeper understanding of methods will also help in evaluating claims, especially competing or contradictory claims. Here, we will review the basic methods used to analyse genes and the genome.

Mutation

Any change in the DNA sequence is a *mutation*, adapted from the Latin word for 'a changing'. Most mutations have no observable effect. Those mutations that do have an effect are typically deleterious. The fact that very few mutations are beneficial probably underlies the pejorative sense

---

Wild-Types and Mutants

A *mutation* is a change in the nucleotide sequence of a DNA molecule, which generates a new allele. The existence of several alleles in a population is called *polymorphism*. The most common sequence is called *wild-type*.

of 'mutant'. However, evolution requires muta-tion, so we are all the descendants of mutants.

Blood group antigens ABO are examples of vari-ations that are all functionally equivalent and all are considered wild-type. An individual may express any combination of A and B antigens or neither (O) on their red cells and be considered normal. These antigens are glycolipids and glyco-proteins against which the immune system can react strongly, which is why it is important to match types for blood transfusions. Their expres-sion depends on the genes encoding the enzymes that synthesize and transfer carbohydrate chains to lipids to proteins.

Types of mutants

Some changes in the genome occur through nat-ural processes, including the movement of DNA segments (transposition) and rearrangement (recombination, crossing over at meiosis). Other mutations occur by chance, such as the misincor-poration of nucleotides during replication, or are induced or increased through exposure to envi-ronmental agents.

DNA mutations may:

• have no effect on the expression of a gene (be silent);
• change the level of gene expression (increase or decrease);
• destroy the protein activity (loss of function);
• create a new protein activity (gain of function);
• produce a structurally different but functionally equivalent protein.

Mutations that change the sequence of an encoded protein are divided into:

• *missense* – encodes a different amino acid;
• *nonsense* – does not encode an amino acid, termi-nating the protein.

DNA can be mutated in various ways:

• *Point mutations* substitute one nucleotide for another;
• *Deletions or insertions* alter both the length and sequence of DNA;
• *Inversions* reverse the order of genes on a chro-mosome;

• *Translocations* move large chromosome pieces within the genome.

Point mutations within coding regions may lead to different amino acids being incorporated into the protein or cause premature termination of transla-tion if a stop codon is introduced (Figure 2.7). Since the genetic code is degenerate (each amino acid is encoded by more than one base triplet), alteration of a single nucleotide may *not* alter the amino acid sequence. The most common point mutation is replacement of cytosine with thymine (C → T, *see* below, *Genes and Methylation*).

Reciprocal deletions and insertions can occur between chromosome pairs as a result of unequal crossing over during meiosis. Deletions from single chromosomes can also occur when a loop forms during DNA replication, which is lost when the two ends reunite (Figure 2.8(a)). Deleted fragments that lack a centromere are lost during subsequent cell divisions. Deletions and insertions range from a single base to several megabases, including whole genes. Small deletions or insertions in the protein-coding portion of a gene usually change the read-ing frame, resulting in *frameshift mutations* and proteins with truncations or dramatically changed sequences (Figure 2.7). Ionizing radiation and mutagenic chemicals increase the spontaneous chromosomal breakage rate.

Inversions occur when a chromosome is broken at two places and the intervening segment is 'flipped' and reinserted back-to-front (Figure 2.8(b)). As with translocations, DNA is not necessarily lost but genes may be disrupted at the breakpoints or brought under control of different regulatory sequences.

Translocations result from the recombination of non-homologous chromosomes or breakage of two chromosomes followed by abnormal repair (Figure 2.8(c)). DNA is not lost or gained during the process. However, if a gene is brought under the control of different regulatory sequence its expression can be dramatically altered. For example, chronic mylogenous leukaemia results from translocating a growth factor gene to a highly transcribed region.

The consequence of a mutation depends on whether it occurs in germ cells or somatic cells.

Silent	Chain termination	Frame shift
Pro Glu Ala Cys Glu	Glu Ala Arg Thr His Leu Ile Asn Gly	Gly Arg Glu Glu Thr Ile Asn Gly Ser
CCC GAG GC**A** TGC GAA	GAG GCC **A**GA ACC CAC CTT ATT AAT GGG	GGG AGG GAG GAA ACG **A**TC AAC GGC AGC
↓	↓	
CCC GAG GC**T** TGC GAA	GAG GCC TGA ACC CAC CTT ATT AAT GGG	GGG AGG GAG GAA ACG TCA ACG GCA GC
Pro Glu Ala Cys Glu	Glu Ala Stop	Gly Arg Glu Glu Thr Ser Thr Ala Ala

Figure 2.7 Small mutations within a protein-coding sequence can dramatically alter the protein. (a) Mutations in the third nucleotide in a codon are often silent, meaning that the protein is not changed. (b) Mutations producing a premature stop codon lead to truncated proteins. (c) Frameshift mutants usually completely change the subsequent amino acids.

Figure 2.8 Chromosome mutations can cause large changes. (a) A chromosome loop can undergo double-stranded break and repair, producing a deletion and a circular piece, which does not have a centromere. (b) A portion of a chromosome can invert. (c) Translocations such as the 'Philadelphia' chromosome, which swaps the ends of chromosomes 9 and 22, causing lymphoma.

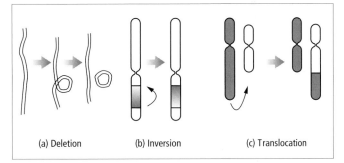

(a) Deletion (b) Inversion (c) Translocation

• Germ cell mutations do not lead to abnormalities in the individual in whom the mutation occurred, but can be inherited and cause disease in subsequent generations.

• Somatic cell mutations in differentiated tissues are not inherited, but may lead to disease in the affected individual. Such mutations are of particular importance in the development of cancer.

Some diseases are always caused by a mutation in one particular gene. The first and best-known example of a point mutation leading to an altered protein product is sickle cell disease, which was shown by V. M. Ingram in 1956 to be caused by altering a single amino acid in the β-globin chain of haemoglobin (Figure 2.9). Haemoglobin is the red blood cell protein that uses iron to bind oxygen in the lungs and release it in peripheral tissues. Such a deleterious mutant should be selected against during evolution, resulting in a low frequency of that allele. However, the abnormal haemoglobin (HbS) that causes sickle cell anaemia in homozygotes may also protect against some consequences of malaria. This may benefit heterozygotes, thereby protecting the allele encoding HbS.

In contrast, many different mutations cause thalassaemias, a group of clinically similar disorders caused by mutations affecting synthesis of alpha or beta haemoglobin subunits. Haemoglobin contains 2 alpha and 2 beta chain subunits. Two genes on chromosome 16 encode the alpha subunits. A single gene on chromosome 11 encodes the beta subunit (Figure 2.10).

Alpha thalassaemia is usually caused by deletions of one or more α-globin genes, although a minority of cases are caused by more subtle mutations. Major deletions in the β-globin genes are rare. Beta thalassaemia is caused by various different point mutations or small deletions in the control regions, reducing transcription, or splice sites, altering mRNA processing, resulting in abnormal, reduced or absent β-globin production (*see* haemoglobinopathies, Chapter 3).

Causes of mutation

Mutations occur spontaneously and can be induced to occur more frequently. Spontaneous mutations result from the biochemistry of

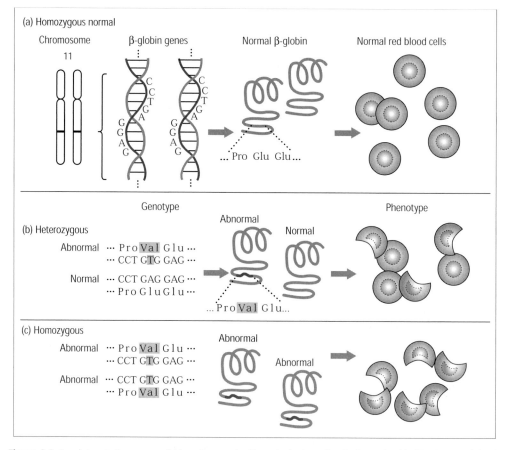

Figure 2.9 A point mutation causes sickle cell anaemia. The substitution of a single nucleotide (GAG → GTG) in the β-globin gene leads to the replacement of glutamic acid with valine. The resulting, abnormal haemoglobin protein (haemoglobin S, HbS) differs in structure. When exposed to low oxygen (hypoxia), which is encountered in the peripheral tissues, the red blood cells (RBCs) containing HbS are prone to dramatic shape changes called sickling. These sickled RBCs are less durable and tend to deteriorate, causing anaemia.

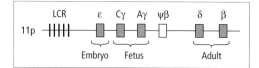

Figure 2.10 The genes of the β-globin family are clustered on the short arm of chromosome 11. The different β-globin genes are ordered in the sequence in which they are expressed during development. Epsilon-globin (ε-globin) is made very early in embryonic development, the two γ-globin variants are expressed during fóetal life, and the delta-(δ-) and β-globin genes take over after birth. A pseudogene is indicated by ψ. The locus control region (LCR) is a group of tissue-specific enhancers that activate transcription in erythroid cells.

nucleotides and replication. Some DNA polymerases are particularly error prone; they are used by cells of the immune system to generate new pathogen receptors (hypermutation). Mutations can also be induced by exposure to chemicals that damage DNA or by viruses that integrate into genomic DNA (proviruses) as part of their life cycle. Although we normally think of chemical mutation as a bad thing, some chemotherapies act through inducing mutations in fast-growing cancer cells.

Spontaneous mutations

Mutations can be caused by copying errors during DNA replication. The main eukaryote DNA polymerases α and δ misincorporate nucleotides at rates ranging from 1 in 50 000 to 1 in 5 million, depending on the nucleotide pair, despite proof-reading activities that correct most mistakes. The most likely misincorporation is the wrong purine or pyrimidine (i.e A ↔ G or T ↔ C). DNA poly-merase can also slip backwards or forwards on the template, causing a duplication or deletion. A fol-low-up editing system called *strand-directed mis-match repair* detects and corrects mismatches in the newly replicated strand, which is identified because it has more breaks in the phosphate backbone between nucleotides (nicks). The 'finished prod-uct', the replicated genome, has about **one error in 1 billion** (E-9). This is thousands-fold better than the 'five nines' (99.999%) accuracy goal of modern manufacturing practice, which equates to one error in one hundred thousand (E-5).

Proofreading is Fundamental

Accurate DNA replication, and specifically proofreading, is so fundamental that it may be the main reason that DNA polymerases work in only the 5' → 3' direction. The energy for DNA synthesis comes from cleavage of deoxynucleotide triphosphates (dNTPs) as they are incor-porated. Like the more familiar energy source adenosine triphosphate (ATP), dNTPs are cleaved to dNp and PP (pyrophosphate). If DNA polymerases *could* extend 3'→ 5' (they cannot), *then* energy would have to come from the triphosphate already on the DNA strand, not the incoming nucleotide. If the last nucleotide was misincor-porated and had to be removed, there would be no energetic triphosphate left at the end of the strand and it could not be extended.

Cytosine nucleotides spontaneously lose an amino group (deamination), yielding uracil. A different repair mechanism, one not linked to replication, corrects the uracil to thymine (U → T).

Both purine and pyrimidine nucleotides can change from their common forms, called the *keto* isomer, to their *enol* isomer. The *enol* form pairs with the wrong base on the other strand, causing a mutation upon replication. A nucleotide can also adopt an imino form instead of the common amino form. An *imino* C pairs with an *amino* A and *vice versa*.

Induced mutations

Chemical mutagens

Agents that cause mutations are called *mutagens*. Mutagens can cause deletion or replacement of the original nucleotide. Chemicals can cause mutations when they:

- insert between nucleotides (intercalate);
- mimic nucleotides (analogues);
- deaminate;
- oxidize;
- alkylate;
- crosslink.

Intercalating agents such as acridine dyes, proflavin or ethidium bromide distort DNA or sta-bilize loops and other single-stranded structures, all of which make DNA polymerase more likely to skip, causing a deletion. Nucleotide analogs, such as bromodeoxyuridine (BrdU), disrupt base pair-ing when they are incorporated. BrdU is a thymine analog that frequently adopts an *enol* form, which pairs with guanine. Hydroxylamine can induce deamination, as can oxidation dam-age. Adenine oxidation yields hypoxanthine, which base pairs with cytosine. Oxidation of gua-nine produces xanthine, which pairs with cyto-sine and so is not a mutation. Mispairing is caused by alkylating agents, such as cyclophosphamide, ethylnitrosourea (ENU), or nitrosoguanidine (NG), and agents that methylate, such as ethane methyl sulphonate (EMS). Chemotherapeutic agents such as platinum (cisplatin) distort DNA and can crosslink DNA to cellular proteins, lead-ing to cell death.

Aflatoxin B1 (AFB1), a product of the fungus *Aspergillus flavus* (mold), is among the most powerful mutagens in nature. The mold and toxin can contaminate certain agricultural crops pre- and post-harvest. AFB1 and benzopyrene, pro-duced by internal combustion engines, are exam-ples of chemical mutagens that form bulky addition products when they bind to DNA.

Radiation damage

Research programmes to understand the deleteri-ous effects of radiation on the genome were begun with the dawn of the atomic age after World War II in England (Harwell) and the United States (Oak Ridge).

- Ultraviolet radiation: UV light from the sun or tanning lamps stimulates the formation of crosslinks between adjacent pyrimidines (*photodimers* and *photoproducts*). Mutations occur when these lesions are repaired improperly.
- Ionizing radiation: Penetrating radiation from cosmic rays, medical X-rays, nuclear waste and radon gas (the most frequent source) produce *reactive oxygen* species including *superoxide radicals* (unpaired electrons) in water. These damage nucleotides and can break DNA strands, producing mutations and even cell death.

Transposition
About half the human genome is composed of DNA sequences that are designed to move (*see* below). DNA at the sites of insertion and excision is mutated in the process. Regulatory sequences, such as promoters and enhancers, and pieces of genes are often carried along with the moving DNA. Shuffling of genomic DNA by transposition was probably crucial in human evolution.

Genome maps

Genetic maps were under construction long before it was known what should be mapped physically. The first maps determined only whether genes were *linked*, that is, close enough to each other to be inherited together. Physical maps began by correlating genetic differences with visible changes on chromosomes. Now, the nucleotide sequence of the entire human genome has been determined.

Linkage maps

It became apparent that genes are arranged linearly soon after T. H. Morgan started mapping fruit fly genes in the early twentieth century. Even the genes on the circular genomes of mitochondria and bacteria can be mapped by linkage. The closer together that two genes lie on the same chromosome, the less likely that they will be separated by a recombination event during meiosis. Therefore, recombination rates can be used to measure distances between genes.

A recombination rate of 1%, 1 crossover in 100, is called a centiMorgan (cM). Two genes separated by 1 cM will be separated by recombination in 1% of meioses. One centiMorgan represents on average about 1 million base pairs of DNA (1 cM ~ 1 Mbp). However, recombination is not random, and thus the actual physical distance represented by a centiMorgan varies according to whether recombination occurs more or less commonly in the region. For example, recombination is higher on the short arms of chromosomes, probably because at least one crossover is necessary for normal disjunction.

Linkage disequilibrium

Some genes are inherited together more often than would be expected by their proximity, a phenomenon called linkage disequilibrium (LD). The suppressed recombination frequency observed in the offspring could result from fewer recombinations at prophase or different survival of the recombinants at some subsequent developmental stage. LD can result if the intergenic chromosomal region does not match homologous chromosomes well, disrupting pairing and suppressing crossing over. Alternatively, LD can result from an interaction between genes. For example, if one protein binds to another, compensatory changes in each protein may render both genes dependent on the other.

Cytogenetics

Cytogenetics is the branch of genetics that studies the overall architecture of chromosomes in cells. It originated with relatively simple but very informative chemical stains and has developed into a sophisticated and powerful molecular tool.

Chromosome banding

Chromosome banding is a way to count chromosomes and assess their structural integrity. It is used to screen for chromosomal changes associated with birth defects and cancer. It is probably the most common genetic test, performed ~500 000 times each year in North America.

- G-banding with Giemsa stain yields the familiar pattern of ~500 light- and dark-stained bands at metaphase (Figure 1.6);
- Q-banding with *q*uinacrine, a fluorochrome, yields a fluorescent pattern very similar to that seen in G-banding;
- C-banding with *b*arium oxide, which stains centromeres and other regions of constitutive heterochromatin (*see* Satellite DNA).
- R-banding (*r*everse-Giemsa stain) is useful for analysing deletions or translocations that involve the telomeres. R-bands are GC-rich regions that remain double stranded and stained after the AT-rich regions are selectively made single stranded (denatured) by heating.
- T-banding is used to stain the *t*elomeric regions after heat denaturation, yielding a subset of R-bands.

Giemsa developed his staining technique in the early twentieth century (Figure 2.11). Fluorescent chromosome banding was introduced in 1969 by Caspersson and Zech. The banding patterns of chromosomes from humans, chimpanzees, gorillas and orangutans are remarkably similar.

Chromatin Stains Reveal Activity

Euchromatin comprises the transcriptionally active regions that stain lightly with basic dyes. *Heterochromatin* comprises the darker staining of chromosomes that are characterized by the presence of condensed chromatin, highly repetitive sequences and relatively low gene density.

Fluorescent *in situ* hybridization

Fluorescent *in situ* hybridization (FISH) localizes genes on chromosomes with light. Probe DNAs, often short synthetic oligonucleotides, are first

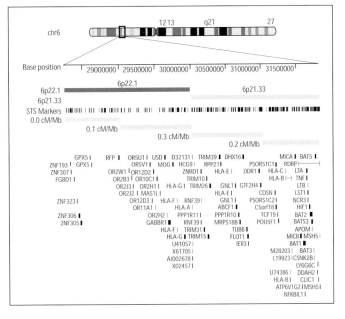

Figure 2.11 Genes are mapped on chromosomes by physical markers and in relation to one another. Three maps of chromosome 6, a chromosome of average length containing ~171 Mb, are shown. (a) An 'ideogram' (symbol) illustrates idealized Giemsa-stained banding patterns. An expanded view of the 6p21–6p22 bands is centred on position 30.02 Mb, approximately the position of the human histocompatibility gene HLA-A. Within this region are shown sequence-tagged sites (STS), recombination rates (cM) and some known genes. This region has low recombination and high linkage disequilibrium. Data were produced by the International Human Genome Sequencing Consortium and interpreted with the genome browser at University of California, Santa Clara (NCBI Build 35, May 2004, genome.ucsc.edu).

labelled with fluorescence and then hybridized to chromosomes (Figure 2.12). Either interphase or spread metaphase (condensed) chromosomes can be hybridized. FISHing with probes from known locations in the genome, such as STSs (*see* below), on interphase chromosomes can resolve genes that are separated by as little as 50 kb. Whole chromosomes can be 'painted' different colours with probes that anneal to chromosome-specific sequences.

FISH extends cytogenetic diagnosis from metaphase to all stages of the cell cycle. Performing FISH when the chromosomes are not condensed, called *interphase cytogenetics*, allows specific genetic rearrangements to be detected without the need for cell culture, thereby greatly accelerating diagnosis. FISH is used in tumour diagnosis. Amplification of the *HER-2/neu* gene on chromosome 17 is associated with poor prognosis in breast cancer. FISH with a *HER-2/neu* probe distinguishes amplified and normal genes.

Comparative genomic hybridization

Comparative genomic hybridization (CGH) finds differences in gene copy number by comparing one genome to another using fluorescence. One genomic DNA, the normal or reference genome, is first amplified and labelled with one colour fluorescent dye. A second genomic DNA, the test genome, often tumour DNA, is amplified and labelled with a second colour fluorescent dye (Figure 2.13). The DNAs are then both added to an unlabelled chromosome. Most genomic regions on the chromosome bind DNAs from both sources, displaying a mixture of colours. However, those regions under- or over-represented in the tumour DNA will be bound preferentially by the reference or tumour DNA, respectively, and appear one colour or the other. Alternatively, the labelled DNA can be hybridized to an *array* of oligonucleotide probes (aCGH). This allows the direct identification of genes deleted or amplified within the test genome.

Molecular analyses using oligonucleotide arrays have revealed that 'normal' chromosomes obtained from healthy people are actually highly variable, carrying numerous small deletions and insertions. These 'large-scale copy-number variants' (LCV) are smaller versions of the previously recognized 'segmental aneuploidies', deletions or duplications ranging upwards from a few chromosome bands. Normal individuals may differ from one another at dozens of LCVs. The notion of a single standard human genome must be abandoned in favour of a normal range of variation.

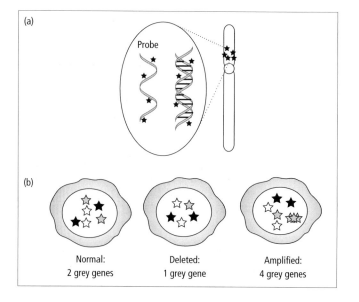

Figure 2.12 Fluorescent *in situ* hybridization (FISH) finds genes on chromosomes. (a) A fluorescent probe hybridizes (base pairs) to a partially denatured target DNA sequence. A condensed, metaphase chromosome is depicted. (b) FISH on interphase chromosomes. Stars filled with white, grey or black represent different colour fluorescent labels binding to DNA within the nucleus of a cell. The cell on left represents two diploid genes (grey and white) and one hemizygous gene (black, one copy). The cell on right represents two diploid white and black genes but amplified grey gene. The actual resolution is much better than suggested by the scale of this diagram.

Figure 2.13 Comparative genomic hybridization detects differences, such as large duplications or deletions, between genomes. The genomic DNAs from the test and reference sources are first labelled with different colour fluorescent dyes and then they are mixed and used as probes in hybridizing to a reference chromosome. Most regions of the genome bind probes from both sources. Those regions deleted or amplified in the test genome preferentially bind the fluorescently labelled reference or test DNA, respectively.

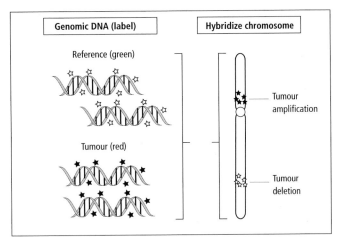

X Chromosome inactivation

In female embryos, one of the two X chromosomes is randomly inactivated in somatic cells. X inactivation does not occur in germ cells. Inactivation occurs on day 16 after fertilization in humans, when the embryo consists of 5000 cells. All these cells' progeny maintain the inactivation of the same X chromosome, which condenses and can often be recognized in female cells as a dark staining 'Barr body' on the edge of the nucleus. Inactivation results in a *mosaic* pattern of expression for some genes on the X chromosome. In heterozygous females, for example, two different allelic forms of the enzyme glucose-6-phosphate dehydrogenase can be detected in large, contiguous patches of different tissues. (X inactivation in female cats occurs at the 64 cell stage and causes similar mosaicism, which can be readily observed in calico coat colour patterns.)

The process of inactivation involves expression of a gene called X-inactivation-specific transcript (*XIST*, 'exist'). XIST, the active gene product, is an RNA, not a protein. Surprisingly, *XIST* is expressed exclusively from the condensed chromosome. Approximately one-fifth of the genes on the 'inactivated' X chromosome are transcribed at normal rates, which may explain why the chromosome disorder Turner syndrome 45, X (single X, no Y), is frequently non-viable in humans (Chapter 3).

X chromosome inactivation may be one mechanism to compensate for the dose effect of some genes on the 2 X chromosomes in females compared to only 1 in males. Consistent with this supposition, females with more than 2 X chromosomes inactivate all but 1. Inactivation is also called *lyonization* after Mary Lyon, the British geneticist who discovered it in 1961.

Physical maps

The DNA from one cell would stretch 2 m if the chromosomes were unpacked and placed end to end. Many different techniques have been developed to analyse these enormous molecules. Analysing genomes often requires cutting the DNA into smaller fragments for sequencing. Determining *where* the fragment belongs in the genome is as important as the sequence itself. Unique sequences or patterns are used as *markers* (landmarks) to orient fragments in the genome.

Chromosome Markers

Markers are genetic sequence variants that serve as chromosomal landmarks.

Southern blot

Southern blot analysis involves separating DNA fragments on a gel, blotting the gel and then hybridizing the blot with a labelled probe

(Figure 2.14). Hybridization is the pairing of a probe sequence with a target sequence based on complementary DNA sequences. The gel separates the DNA fragments according to size and hybridization detects specific sequences, allowing the identification of DNA fragments. For example, to determine the size of the genomic *Eco*RI fragment(s) containing the β-globin gene, one would cut genomic DNA with *Eco*RI, separate the fragments on a gel, blot and probe with a fragment of the β-globin gene. Alternatively, to test whether a polymerase chain reaction (PCR)-amplified product is what you think it is, you might blot it and probe the blot with a labelled fragment of the gene.

An important application of Southern blotting is in pedigree analysis (Figure 2.14). This tests whether offspring carry particular alleles. Alleles are distinguished by either the fragment sizes or hybridization strengths. Phenotypes may change dramatically in a generation despite the similar allele frequency. In this example, the homozygous

offspring may gain or lose traits compared to their heterozygous parents.

Restriction fragment length polymorphism

A powerful, widely used method of identifying genetic differences is restriction fragment length polymorphism (RFLP). DNA treated with a restriction endonuclease is cut at specific sequences or *restriction sites*. In the case of genomic DNA, this produces a large number of *restriction fragments* of many different lengths. Any changes in the sequence within the restriction site, which would block cutting, or changes in the distance between restriction sites, such as the number of repetitive sequences, changes the restriction fragment length. Thus, RFLP is a sensitive measure of genetic variation between two individuals (Figure 2.15). RFLPs were used to map on chromosome 7 the CFTR gene, which when mutant causes cystic fibrosis.

Repetitive sequences 1 – satellite DNA

Repeat sequences comprise an estimated 45% of the human genome and have no known function.

> **Southern Blots Identity DNA**
>
> A Southern blot is performed to identify and to determine the size of a DNA fragment.

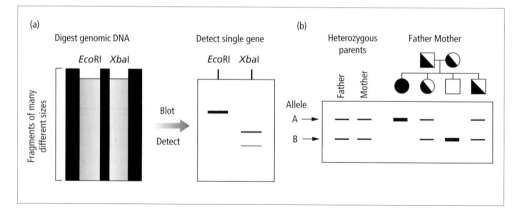

Figure 2.14 Southern blots analyse DNA sequences. (a) In this example, genomic DNA is first digested with restriction enzymes and the many different-sized fragments are separated on a gel. The gel is then blotted and the gene is detected by hybridization to a labelled probe. Here, the gene is found on one *Eco*RI fragment and two smaller *Xba*I fragments, meaning that the gene is flanked by *Eco*RI sites and there is an *Xba*I site within the gene. (b) Southern blots can help in pedigree analysis. In this example, digestion of genomic DNA with a restriction enzyme produces different-sized fragments. This is known as restriction fragment length polymorphism (RFLP). If the larger fragment (indicated with black in the pedigree) were associated with a disease, such an analysis would strongly suggest close monitoring of the first offspring (the daughter represented by a filled circle). The second and fourth offspring are heterozygous carriers of the disease-associated gene and the third offspring does not carry the disease-associated allele (the son represented by an open square).

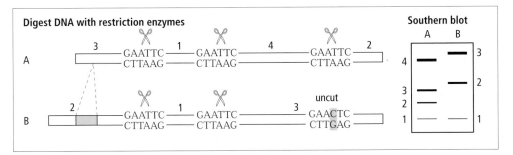

Figure 2.15 Genetic variations can be identified by RFLP. DNA is digested with a restriction endonuclease (here, *Eco*RI), then Southern blotted. The DNAs labelled A and B differ in two ways: A has three restriction sites while B has two, and an insertion (or deletion) has occurred within one fragment. These differences are reflected in the pattern of bands on the Southern blot. Although several bands are shown on the Southern blot, typically only a single gene would be detected with a labelled probe.

Table 2.1 Several types of repeated sequences are found in the human genome.

	Repeat name	Repeat size (bp)	Total size (kb)	Features
1	Satellite	5–200	<100	Found in heterochromatin and centromeres. Not transcribed
2	Minisatellite			
	Hypervariable family	10–60	1–20	Common core sequence GGGCAGGANG,
		6	1–20	dispersed, VNTRs usually TTAGGG and
	Telomeric family			repeated about a thousand times. Protects chromosome ends
3	Microsatellite	1–4	<1	Repeats of A and CA are the most common. Dispersed throughout genome

Abbreviations: bp, base pairs; kb, thousand bp; VNTRs, variable numbers of tandem repeats.

They form large arrays that were originally called *satellites* because they form a minor peak upon density separation due to their content of G–C nucleotides. Several different types of repeat sequences have been characterized (Table 2.1).

Satellite DNA is typically not transcribed and forms the bulk of heterochromatin (chromatin that remains condensed during interphase). The *hypervariable* family of minisatellite DNA shares a sequence motif and is dispersed. The number of these repeats at any given locus varies, thereby forming one method of identification called *variable numbers of tandem repeats* (VNTRs). The *telomeric* family of minisatellite DNA almost certainly protects the chromosome ends from random recombination events. Microsatellite DNA consists of runs of dinucleotide repeats, most commonly

CA (or TG on the complementary strand), that are dispersed throughout the genome. Microsatellite repeats are found throughout the genome, a characteristic that contributed to them becoming a favoured marker in gene mapping.

Variations in the number of minisatellite repeats between individuals can be detected by using a restriction enzyme that cuts outside an array of repeats. These variations give rise to different-sized DNA fragments, which can be separated in a gel and detected by hybridization with a probe that recognizes the repetitive unit. With the exception of identical twins, there are variations in minisatellite regions between all individuals and these variable regions are inherited in a Mendelian fashion. This forms the basis for the technique of *DNA fingerprinting*, in which the sizes of minisatellite regions at numerous loci are determined by probing restriction fragments of total DNA.

Highly repeated DNA sequences are thought to form when DNA polymerase slips during DNA replication. Slipping occurs more frequently when copying a repeated region, hence, repeats can accumulate rapidly through generations. Large changes in repeat numbers can occur quickly through unequal crossing over, which is more likely in repeat regions because the homologous chromosomes can efficiently pair anywhere along the repeated region.

Genes and methylation – CpG islands

Potential genes can be identified within large pieces of DNA by looking for CpG 'islands', which are often found at the 5′ end of genes. The dinucleotide CpG occurs only about one-fifth as often as expected from the frequency of C and G (0.21×0.21). This is because CpG is usually methylated in mammalian genomes. Methylated CpG undergoes spontaneous deamination, yielding UpG dinucleotides that are repaired to TpG. However, the CpG dinucleotides lying near actively transcribed genes are usually unmethylated, so they are protected from this transition.

Certain unmethylated CpGs can be readily identified because they are cut by the restriction enzyme *Hpa*II ('hoppa 2′), which recognizes the sequence CCGG when the Cs are unmethylated. Since CpGs near genes tend to be unmethylated, *Hpa*II cuts genomic DNA much more frequently near active genes, producing '*Hpa*II tiny fragments'. Methylation patterns are lost when DNA is cloned in bacteria, so the screen must be performed directly on genomic DNA prepared from mammalian cells. Yeast, also a eukaryote, and fruit flies (*Drosophila*) do not methylate their genomes and rely on different mechanisms for regulating gene expression.

The mammalian immune system utilizes the methylation differences between some eukaryotes and prokaryotes. Certain proteins on leukocytes bind the CpGs in bacterial genomes, which are never methylated (accounting for the higher CG content of prokaryote genomes). These binding proteins provide extra stimulation to the leukocytes defending against a bacterial infection.

Somatic cell hybridization – radiation hybrid mapping

One method for localizing genes to particular chromosomes is *somatic cell hybridization*. This technique exploits the fact that when cells from different species are fused, the resulting hybrid cells randomly lose chromosomes. This can produce cells in which only particular human chromosomes are present. These cells can then be screened for the presence of either a known DNA sequence (using a labelled cloned DNA fragment), or the protein product of a specific gene. Alternatively, the donor cell can be irradiated, which causes chromosomal breakage.

Radiation hybrids (RH) are created when chromosomal fragments, generated by irradiation of one cell type, are allowed to integrate into the chromosomes of a second cell type, often a cell from a different species. Many RH are mouse cells that retained one human chromosome after fusion with human cells. This technique provided much information about the physical location of genes at the beginning of genomic research and is still used for mapping.

Expressed sequence tag – transcript maps

The most information-rich part of the genome consists the genes that encode messenger RNA (mRNA). These comprise only a small part of the genome (*see* accounting below) and they can be found relatively easily by starting with the RNA and working back to the gene (*see* cDNA, p 35). A comprehensive effort to sequence all mRNAs, in the form of cDNAs, was started in the early 1990s. All of the cDNA clones obtained from a particular tissue represent a library of the genes that were expressed when the tissue was obtained. In 1994, an international consortium was formed to construct a physical human gene map of cDNA-based, *expressed sequence tag* (EST, 'ee-ess-tee') markers. ESTs are short, unique sequences of cDNA. By 1998 a map of 30 181 human gene-based EST markers had been assembled and integrated with genetic maps produced by radiation hybrid mapping. This map includes most genes that encode proteins of known function.

Sequence-tagged site – genome landmark

A good map has many easily identified landmarks. Such reference points on the map of the human genome are provided by sequence-tagged sites (STSs). STSs are unique sequences in the genome that can be amplified by PCR. (PCR is a fundamental tool in genetic analysis that is explained in detail in Chapter 1.) They serve as markers in genetic mapping, allowing smaller pieces of DNA to be aligned and combined into larger physical maps. Conditions for PCR amplification of STSs, including the primer sequences, buffers and temperatures, are available on the internet. For example, over 3000 STSs are defined for the ~180 Mbp of chromosome 6, an average of one STS per 60 kb.

Artificial chromosomes – bacterial and yeast

Plasmids are excellent for cloning a few kilobases of DNA (*see* Chapter 1). Cosmids are very large plasmids that can be used for cloning larger fragments (up to 45 kb). Cosmids also contain *cos* sites (*cohesive* sequences), which allows them to be packaged into *bacteriophage* particles for more efficient subcloning and identification (bacteriophages infect bacteria).

Limitations on the size of DNA fragments that can be cloned into vectors have been overcome by incorporating large fragments of human DNA into *yeast artificial chromosomes* (YACs). Complete genomic DNA libraries were created by fractionating human chromosomes, inserting fragments of up to 2 million bp in length into YACs, and growing them in yeast (*Saccharomyces cerevisiae*). Later, the development of bacterial artificial chromosomes (BACs) facilitated completion of the Human Genome Project. BACs are propagated as stable inserts in bacteria (*Escherichia coli*), and are

usually about 150 kbp in length. A database of the sequences of the ends of BAC clones has been created, providing a framework to link DNA sequences over large regions. These DNA libraries can then be used to create physical maps of *contiguous* sequences (contigs) of human chromosomes. BACs have superseded YACs for most large cloning efforts.

Libraries are Complex Collections

A *library* is a collection of clones, usually mixed together. Each clone represents a small part of a complex whole.

Finding genes – forward and reverse genetics, positional cloning

If the DNA sequence of the gene is known, then the gene can be physically mapped to a specific chromosomal region by a process known as *forward genetics*. Until recently, this would involve cloning larger regions of chromosomal DNA, which would be sequenced and positioned by looking for STSs. Now, the cloned sequence is simply compared to the sequence of the entire human genome. Query sequences can be submitted over the internet to powerful computer programs (e.g. BLAST, *basic local alignment search tool*) that quickly search the genome databases (e.g. GenBank or EMBL) and return a region or regions of sequence match.

If the only information about a gene is the physical characteristic (phenotype) it produces, then the gene can be mapped by a process known as *reverse genetics*. This approach is based on linkage analysis using panel of a genomic markers, which is established through pedigree analysis using molecular tools such as RFLP, STSs and *single nucleotide polymorphisms* (SNPs, *see* below). The strength of linkage (probability) is measured by LOD (*logarithm of the odds*) score.

Cloning a gene based on its location is known as *positional cloning*. The region of interest can be examined for evidence of functional genes. Candidate genes are identified, cloned and sequenced. The amino acid sequence of the protein product can be deduced and the cloned gene can be expressed in an artificial expression system. It is necessary to confirm that the candidate disease gene is found in affected individuals.

Experimental animal models are invaluable tools to determining the function of genes. For example, if a mutant gene causes a similar disease in mice, it constitutes nearly unassailable proof of causality and provides an excellent experimental setting to identify and test preclinical therapies.

Applications of PCR in genetic analysis

In whole genomes PCR can be used to find polymorphisms, identify new mutations in smaller regions or test for even a single nucleotide change.

For known mutants, primers may be designed to either *overlie* or *flank* the mutation. An overlying primer is designed to match either the common, wild-type sequence or a mutation. If the primer matches the common DNA sequence, amplification will occur with DNA from normal individuals. If the primer matches the mutated sequence, amplification occurs with DNA from affected individuals. Flanking primers amplify both mutant and wild-type template sequences. The DNA amplification product (also called an 'amplicon') can then be analysed for the mutation using a separate procedure.

Amplification refractory mutation system

Single nucleotide differences can be resolved in PCR (Figure 2.16). This key method relies on the fact that DNA polymerase extends a complementary strand very quickly but pauses a relatively long time before extending a strand with even a single nucleotide mismatch at the 3' end. By exploiting this difference in speed, normal and mutant alleles may be easily distinguished. If primer is designed to match the wild-type allele, then amplicons rapidly accumulate in the presence of sample DNA with the wild-type, but not the mutant, allele sequence.

Whole genome amplification

Although any single test usually requires only a small amount of DNA, investigators often want to perform many different tests with a limited amount of original sample. For example, very small amounts of irreplaceable DNA may be recovered from valuable sources, such as stored blood samples or early embryos.

Three amplification methods are in use:

1 Degenerate oligonucleotide primed PCR (DOP-PCR) relies on the extension of randomly annealed primers. This technique does not

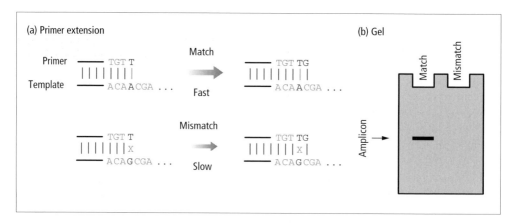

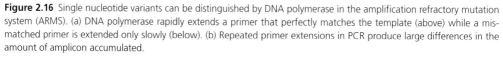

Figure 2.16 Single nucleotide variants can be distinguished by DNA polymerase in the amplification refractory mutation system (ARMS). (a) DNA polymerase rapidly extends a primer that perfectly matches the template (above) while a mismatched primer is extended only slowly (below). (b) Repeated primer extensions in PCR produce large differences in the amount of amplicon accumulated.

amplify the genome uniformly, generating instead over- and under-represented regions.

2 'GenomePlex' randomly digests the DNA template then uses a proprietary (company secret) process to convert the ends into universal priming sites. This method amplifies uniformly ~1000 fold.

3 Multiple displacement amplification (MDA), like DOP-PCR, extends randomly annealed primers. MDA uses a special DNA polymerase, derived from a bacteriophage (phi29), that makes very long products and tends to displace, rather than degrade, the complementary strand. This method amplifies uniformly several thousandfold.

Amplification has its limits. Nanogram amounts of genomic DNA produce good representation in the amplified material. One diploid human genome contains ~7 pg DNA, so 1 ng (1000 pg) of starting DNA sample contains ~140 copies of the genome. If one were to amplify much less than 1 ng, there might be too few DNA molecules and statistical effects must be considered. For example, 1 pg of DNA could only represent about 15% of a single genome.

Human genome – why are we similar and how do we differ?

Genomics, the study of genomes, asks big questions about gene expression, variation and evolution. What are the genetic differences among humans? How did differences occur and propagate? What are the genetic differences that separate humans from non-human primates or other animals? Genomics has expanded greatly in the last 20 years as new technologies in chromosome analysis and especially in DNA sequencing grew more powerful.

Human genomics will be the key to finding disease-causing genes and molecular pathways. Pathogen genomics has already found alleles underlying virulence differences and helped to design therapy. The accumulation of genetic knowledge suggests that physicians will be increasingly able to use the patient's own genome to guide treatment – the promise of personalized medicine.

Human Genome Project – sequence

Collaborative efforts of over 100 laboratories resulted in the 1994 publication of the first high-resolution, comprehensive human linkage map. It consisted of 5840 loci with an average distance of 0.7 cM between them. These markers were mostly microsatellites but included STSs and single nucleotide polymorphisms (SNPs). This map served as a scaffold for organizing the sequencing efforts. Sequencing of different regions was coordinated between laboratories to avoid duplicating work.

The International Human Genome Sequencing Consortium released in 2001 a 'working draft' of the human genome sequence, ~3.1 thousand million (3.1×10^9) bp representing the vast majority of our genetic blueprint. The Consortium included scientists at 20 centres in China, France, Germany, Japan, the United Kingdom, and the United States. They used many different techniques and encouraged the development of new ones. The demands of analysis also promoted the development of computer tools. Although the entire sequence is freely available on the Internet, its value is greatly increased by the analytical and display tools available online at the different centres (e.g. ncbi.nih.gov, sanger.ac.uk, ensembl.org). If the entire human genome sequence were printed in this typeface, it would stretch nearly from London to Los Angeles (and back, if diploid!).

Human Genome: DNA and Genes
The haploid human genome is ~3 100 000 000 nucleotides, which encode ~23 000 protein-coding genes.

A private company named Celera Genomics assembled its own version of the human genome sequence, which was made fully available only to subscribers. Celera used a different approach called Whole Genome Assembly (described below). The private effort initially relied on publicly available genomic scaffolds to organize and orient their sequences. An estimated 60% of the sequence itself also came from the public project.

Competition between the public and private sequencing efforts spurred innovation and accelerated analysis.

Final version

The final version of the genome sequence was released late in 2004 ('build' 35). This sequence excludes heterochromatin because it contains many repetitive sequences and few single copy genes and is very hard to sequence. The final sequence covers 99% of the euchromatin and contains 2.85 billion nucleotides. It is 99.999% accurate (estimated 1 error in 100 000 bases). Many of the remaining 341 gaps are associated with duplications and will probably require new sequencing methods to close. The sequence has been an invaluable aid to identifying human genes and understanding how they are organized and regulated.

Whole genome assembly

The newest method of genome analysis is simple in principle but difficult in practice. In WGA, huge numbers of random clones are sequenced ('shotgun') then the sequence overlaps are identified by computer and used to reconstruct the whole genome. This method was enabled by robotic cloning, more efficient sequencing reactions that produce longer 'reads', and improved computing applications. First employed on a large genome by Celera, this method is now refined and used routinely by many groups for sequencing most new genomes for which scaffolds are not available. The relatively small genomes of pathogens are now routinely sequenced by WGA. WGA can be very quick since it dispenses with a preliminary scaffold or mapping. This is a particular advantage in public health emergencies. [Acronym warning – 'WGA' is used for whole genome *assembly, amplification*, or (most commonly) association.]

The 'human instruction book' – decoding needed

The genome sequence is not a catalogue of genes. It has *very* long strings of the 4 bases (ATGC) with little clear punctuation, containing overlapping 'words' mixed with large amounts of apparently meaningless 'junk'. This complex code is being solved slowly, revealing a great deal about human physiology and history.

The joint government statement on the completion of the human genome sequence called it the 'molecular instruction book of human life'. Let's compare it to a more familiar book, for example, the Encyclopaedia Britannica, which contains in its eleventh edition 44 million words. This amounts to probably ~300 million letters, about one-tenth the number of nucleotides in the entire human genome. However, DNA has only 4 'letters', far fewer than the English alphabet's 26, even without considering punctuation, numbers and case. Consequently, the Encyclopaedia *could* contain much more information than the human genome ($26\wedge3E8 > 4\wedge3E9$). Clearly, genomic information is very compactly coded.

Interpreting the genome sequence remains a challenge but certain conclusions can be drawn. For example, investigators report that there are ~23 000 protein-coding genes, which comprise about 1% of the genome (*see* Table 2.2). They arrived at that number by searching the sequence for certain characteristics of known protein-coding genes, such as ORFs (*open reading frames*, a transcript that is not interrupted by stop codons) and TATA sequences upstream (which can specify where transcription starts), and then comparing the putative protein with previously identified transcripts, many of them EST clones (*see expressed sequence tag*, above). To appreciate the challenge of gene identification, consider the clotting factor VIII. Mutations in factor VIII cause haemophilia A (*see* Chapter 3). Its coding sequence comprises less than 3% of the contiguous genomic sequence because it is encoded by 26 relatively small exons spanning 200 kb of DNA. The dystrophin gene (p 112) spans 2.4 Mb and the titin gene has 363 exons. Given their large genomic size, it is uncertain that these genes would be identified by sequence analysis alone. Indeed, a recent comprehensive analysis using oligonucleotides representing the entire non-repetitive sequence of the human genome identified over 10 000 transcripts that were not among the known or predicted genes. These probably include micro RNAs whose functions are beginning to be elucidated.

Table 2.2 Composition of the human genome.

Genome	Description
45%	Repeats (transposons, etc.)
5%	Segmental duplications
3%	Micro- and minisatellite
1%	Protein coding (exons)
1%	tRNA and rRNA

Duplications are large (10–50 kb), highly homologous regions found on the same or different chromosome. The remaining portion of the genome may be 'junk', largely transposon fragments that have diverged beyond recognition (*see* below).

Titin has 363 Exons

Titin is a huge protein with a spring-like structure that helps give muscle its elastic recoil. It is found in skeletal and heart muscle and mutations in the titin gene have been implicated in certain forms of muscular dystrophy and cardiomyopathy (disease of heart muscle).

Repetitive sequences 2 – Transposons and 'junk'

About half the human genome is repeat sequences. Some repeated sequences have clear functions. For example, ribosomal RNA genes are repeated up to 2000 times (5S subunit) and transfer RNA genes are repeated with only small changes ~1300 times. Others derive from movable sequences called transposable elements, or *transposons*. They are classified as long interspersed nuclear elements (LINEs), short interspersed nuclear elements (SINEs), long terminal repeat (LTR) retrotransposons, or DNA transposons (Table 2.3, Transposons). The first three move through an RNA product; DNA transposons encode an enzyme (transposase) that performs excision and integration (cut and paste) when the element moves.

Large families of repeated sequences were expected from earlier physical studies that analysed the refolding of melted DNA. One family of repeats was recognized early: *Alu*, the major subset of SINEs in humans.

The expansion of transposon families is largely attributable to their intrinsic ability to propagate and not to any advantage to the host. However,

Table 2.3 Mobile DNA sequences comprise a large part of the human genome.

Transposon	Genome	Transmission	Characteristics	Notes
LINEs	21%	RNA, vertical	RNAP II transcript, encodes endonuclease and reverse transcriptase (RT)	6–8 kb; Many truncated 'dead' fragments
SINEs	13%	RNA, vertical	Flanked by direct repeats; RNAP III transcribed, no protein	100–300 bp; Many *Alu* elements; require LINE RT to move (parasitic)
LTR retrotransposons	8%	RNA, horizontal and vertical	Flanked by long terminal (direct) repeats (LTR), some encode protease, RT, RNase H and integrase	6–11 kb; Can acquire, envelope and become exogenous retrovirus; Many single LTR fragments
DNA transposon	3%	DNA, horizontal	Inverted repeats; encodes cut-and-paste transposase	2–3 kb; Many 'dead' fragments compete for transposase

RNA polymerase II (RNAP II) transcribes most protein-coding genes; RNAP III transcribes tRNA and rRNA genes. Vertical transmission is to direct descendants in the next generation, horizontal transmission is to other humans (e.g. through blood transfusion) and other animals. Size refers to the intact transposon; many smaller, inactive fragments litter the human genome.

Repeats may have Functions

Alu elements are short (~300 bp), moderately repetitive (500 000 copies) dispersed sequences that contain a site recognized by the restriction enzyme *Alu* I. Oddly, the *Alu* element derived from an RNA portion of the signal recognition particle, which helps new proteins move out of the cell. *Alu* repeats may contribute to genomic replication and promote recombination. For example, recombination between *Alu* repeats in the cholesterol receptor gene causes deletions, resulting in familial hypercholesterolaemia (Chapter 3, p 95).

---

even these parasitic or 'selfish' genes shuffle regulatory sequences, generating new gene expression patterns. Investigators have also identified 43 genes that probably originated as DNA transposons, including the recombinases that generate diversity in the immune system (RAG1 and RAG2).

Species similarity – why are we similar?

No single human possesses a genome that matches 'the' human genome sequence. Instead, the sequence is a mosaic of sequences from many different humans. Various techniques, more imaginative and less expensive than simply sequencing many different human genomes, have allowed comparisons among humans and between species.

Gene families – copy, edit, repeat

Genes with similar structure and function (gene families) occur throughout the human genome. Genes that are similar are often said to be *homologous*. Strictly speaking, homology implies an evolutionary link between two or more genes or proteins. Homologous proteins that perform the same function in different species are called *orthologues*, while those that perform different but related functions in one species are called *paralogues*.

Gene families may be clustered together, such as the five beta-like globin genes on chromosome 11 (Figure 2.10) or dispersed throughout the genome (e.g. ribosomal RNA (rRNA) genes are found on five different chromosomes). Histone genes are clustered at a few locations on chromosomes 1, 6 and 12. Gene families often contain pseudogenes

(ψ), which are similar in structure to functional members of the gene family but are themselves inactive because of alterations in their regulatory sequences, coding regions or both. The variety and importance of gene families suggests that the human genome has evolved through successive gene duplications and mutations.

Although evolution leads to the accumulation of many differences, the human genome contains DNA sequences that are closely related to those of other species. These DNA sequences appear to have been 'conserved' during the process of evolution. For example, genes encoding histone proteins are remarkably similar in different species. Scientists report that there are nearly 500 sequences of over 200 bp that are absolutely conserved (100% identical) between the orthologous regions of human, rat and mouse genomes. Another 5000 sequences of over 100 bp are absolutely conserved among these species.

Human geno.me structure – history and population growth

The history of human development has defined the pattern of genetics in the world today. All 6 billion humans living on earth today are thought to descend from about 10 000 individuals living about 75 000 years ago in Africa. This population explosion has consequences for the human gene pool:
- Close genetic relatedness (one species)
- Shared set of genetic difference (common SNPs)
- Clustered gene inheritance (haplotypes).

People are genetically very similar. On average, two unrelated people differ at only one nucleotide in one thousand. In other words, people are 99.9% identical. While this 0.1% difference seems negligible, it corresponds to millions of nucleotides (0.1% of $3 \times 10^9 = 3$ million) and accounts for much human variation. Less obviously, these differences can combine to produce enormous differences in health.

Single nucleotide polymorphisms

Single nucleotide polymorphisms (SNPs) are on nucleotides that *differ* among people. In early

2003, the Human Genome Project released a database with 3.7 million SNPs. Using SNPs greatly improves the efficiency of comparing genomes by avoiding the analysis of largely identical sequences. Additional SNPs are now deposited in the public database of SNPs (dbSNP). Particularly valuable are the *reference SNP* ('rs'), which enable extremely rapid and robust mapping. Different laboratories can compare results using these well-documented reference SNPS. For example, rs4949 (Table 2.4) is used to diagnose FRAXA.

Table 2.4 International Union of Pure and Applied Chemistry (IUPAC) code of nucleotide symbols permit simple, unambiguous descriptions of genetic variations. For example, the C/T SNP within the reference sequence #4949 (rs4949) can be shown as: TATAAGAGACACA-GAATCATAAATGYTTTTGCATTTGGAAAATGTACATCC.

Code	Meaning	Mnemonic
A	Adenine	
C	Cytosine	
G	Guanine	
T	Thymine	
U	Uracil (RNA)	
R	A or G	puRine
Y	C or T	pYrimidine
W	A or T	Weak bond
S	C or G	Strong bond
M	A or C	aMino
K	G or T	Keto
B	C or G or T	not A
D	A or G or T	not C
H	A or C or T	not G
V	A or C or G	not T or U
N	G or A or T or C	aNy

All human populations worldwide share the SNPs present in the small, original population. SNPs arising later in human population expansion are unique to different sub-populations. There are about 10 million SNPs possessed by at least 1% of humans. These relatively common SNPs are the focus of most current investigations. In tests, SNPs have proven capable of locating genes involved in several diseases, including sickle cell anaemia, psoriasis, migraine, Alzheimer and diabetes.

Haplotypes – disease susceptibility and drug interactions

Despite the efficiency of SNPs, analysing millions of nucleotides is daunting. Fortunately for the gene mappers, these millions of nucleotide variations do not all segregate independently. Instead, many are inherited together in blocks known as haplotypes (Figure 2.17). Haplotypes are a more systematic way of analysing gene linkage, as stretches of genome instead of individual genes. More than 80% of the genome falls into segments of near complete linkage disequilibrium (LD). Although haplotypes can speed initial mapping, they slow fine mapping and gene identification because the low recombination rate makes it hard to separate candidate disease genes.

Haplotype Blocks
A haplotype is a 5–100 kb length of DNA unbroken by recombination.

Human haplotype map – HapMap

The goal of the international human haplotype mapping (HapMap) project is to identify common human haplotypes (www.hapmap.org). The map is expected to accelerate the discovery of genes related to common diseases, such as asthma, cancer, diabetes and heart disease. Certain SNPs that are found to be usually associated with a particular haplotype then can be used to quickly identify that haplotype. Ideally, one SNP will represent tens of thousands of nucleotides, accelerating analysis enormously.

Preliminary analyses of haplotypes in human populations around the world indicated that a more comprehensive haplotype survey of four populations would be particularly valuable. The tag SNPs for the HapMap were developed from information obtained from 270 individuals from these 4 populations (Table 2.5).

The first draft of the HapMap, consisting of 1 million SNPs, was released to the public in February 2005. Compared with testing all of the currently known 10 million SNPs, this represents a 10- to 50-fold saving of time and money. Depending on

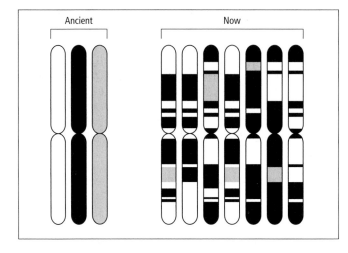

Figure 2.17 Genomes evolve with recombination 'hotspots' separating blocks of DNA called haplotypes. The block pattern represents regions of DNA derived from the same chromosome, not cytogenetic banding patterns. Here, modern haplotypes are formed from recombinations of 3 ancient chromosomes, generating a mosaic pattern. For simplicity, the mosaic pattern of the ancient chromosomes and the many small mutations that would have accumulated on the modern chromosomes are not shown.

Table 2.5 Populations from several countries were analysed for the original HapMap.

Location	Samples
Ibadan, Nigeria	90 from 30 trios (both parents and child) of Yorba ancestry
United States	90 from 30 trios of northern and western European ancestry
Tokyo, Japan	45 unrelated individuals
Beijing, China	45 unrelated individuals of Han ancestry
Worldwide	**270 people**

what the HapMap ultimately tells us, it may prove necessary to analyse fewer than 100-thousand SNPs to provide important clinical information for personalized medicine. This would certainly speed the adoption and implementation of genome-based medicine. Determining exactly *which* SNPs are most valuable is a goal of current research.

Surprisingly, haplotypes are *not* conserved between humans and our nearest evolutionary relative, chimpanzees, despite our genome sequences being 99% identical. Recombination may be dictated more by changes such as methylation, acetylation and other so-called *epigenetic* factors, than by the underlying sequence. This underscores the importance of genomic structure in determining the evolution of species.

Population diversity – how do we differ?

Although the human genome can be recognized as a distinct set of chromosomes with specific sizes and banding patterns, the DNA sequences and their organization is continually changing. Errors introduced during DNA replication, during both meiosis and mitosis, contribute to diversity. Perhaps more important, the combinations of alleles changes in each generation. The allele frequency also changes, albeit slowly, in a population over time. A firm, mathematical foundation for understanding how populations of genomes change over time was established before it was known that genes were made of DNA (e.g. Hardy–Weinberg).

Disease – linkage and association studies

Mendelian disorders are caused by single gene mutations, many of which have been identified (Chapter 3). For most common diseases including cancer, cardiovascular disease, diabetes and autoimmunity, many genes and environmental factors combine to cause or influence the course of disease. These are called *polygenic or multifactorial* diseases. As more diseases are linked to specific genes or combinations of genes, the value in finding these disease alleles will increase (*see* also Chapter 3, Polygenic Disorders).

The influence of genes and the environment can be estimated from disease *concordance*, the incidence of disease among siblings. Identical (monozygotic) twins are especially informative. For a genetically determined disease such as cystic fibrosis, both the identical twins or neither twin will suffer the disease (100% concordance). In contrast, if one identical twin develops the autoimmune disease systemic lupus erythematosus (SLE, lupus), the other twin will develop lupus in about one-half of the cases. This high concordance suggests that genes contribute to, but do not determine, the occurrence of SLE. Concordance for SLE between fraternal twins (non-identical, dizygotic) is much lower, about 1 in 20 (5%). This incidence is higher than the general population, probably because fraternal twins share many genes and environmental exposures. The chance that any sibling of an affected person will be also affected is called the sibling risk ratio (λ_S, 'lambda S'). For SLE, a sibling of an affected is about 25 times more likely to develop the disease ($\lambda_S \sim 25$).

Linkage analysis

Linkage analysis identifies the chromosomal location of gene variants influencing a disease. This analysis was invented for finding dominant genes using families with more than one affected member ('multiplex' families). Subsequent modifications permitted the identification of recessive genes using two or more affected siblings ('affected sib pair'). DNA samples from these family members are tested for shared genes using a very large number of markers (variants) chosen because they are evenly spread over the entire genome. Whereas markers that are not associated with the disease are only randomly shared between the affected and unaffected family members, markers that are closely linked to the genes influencing the disease will be found much more often in members with the disease. The statistical analysis of linkage produces a measurement usually expressed as a logarithm of the odds, or LOD score. A LOD score over 3.6 (equivalent to approximately 1 : 4000 odds) is generally considered to be a strong indication that the observed correlation is caused by real linkage instead of chance.

Genetic Linkage vs. Disease Association

Disease genes are found in linkage and association studies. Linkage defines the relationship between two genes. Association defines statistical coincidence, such as an allele and a disease.

Linkage analysis has been very successful in finding single gene variants that cause disorders (monogenic). For diseases caused by multiple genes, however, linkage analysis is much more difficult. It is especially difficult to assemble the necessary multiplex families when the disease onset is later in life, such as common forms of cardiovascular disease or Alzheimer disease, because fewer members of the earlier generations survive to contribute DNA or clinical data.

A company named deCODE identifies disease genes using genomic and medical data from over half the adult population of Iceland, over 100 000 individuals. These analyses are aided by genealogical information stretching back over a millennium to a small number of founders. This relatively homogeneous genetic composition speeds analysis but raises the question of whether the findings will be applicable to wider populations. Nevertheless, the identified genes tell us something important about the physiology of disease.

Association studies

Association studies determine the frequency of particular genetic markers, usually among unrelated individuals. Since these studies do not require the recruitment of entire families, it is easier to enroll more affected and unaffected (control) individuals. Also, the statistical power of association studies is greater because there is less chance of sharing unrelated genes. However, association is not sufficient to demonstrate cause. The associated gene may lie very close to the gene that actually causes the disorder.

Personalized medicine – pharmacogenomics

Genes may help us understand why some medicines only benefit some people and can harm others – the field of pharmacogenomics. Genetic screening is already entering the clinic, promising to spare patients and physicians the long wait to see whether a newly prescribed drug will be effective. (Note that such genetic screening does not currently help address the dangerous sensitivities that result from particular exposures, such as penicillin allergies, and usually involve more complicated genetic influences.)

The cancer drug gefitinib (trade name Iressa, similar to Tarceva) illustrates the promise and challenge of personalized medicine. In a clinical trial with over one thousand patients with advanced non-small-cell lung cancer, most showed no response to gefitinib; however, about 1 in 10 showed impressive improvement. Gefitinin targets a tyrosine kinase portion of the epidermal growth factor receptor (EGFR), which is often overexpressed on cancer cells. Normally, growth factors bind the EGFR and activate the kinase, causing the cells to grow, divide and spread. Among the drug responders, an EGFR mutation was found in 15 out of 18 patients but very few mutations were detected in unresponsive patients. This finding suggests that a simple screen could identify those patients who would benefit from the drug, although more patients must be analysed in such detail to test this suggestion. These findings also demonstrate the importance of understanding the molecular mechanism of a drug activity before engaging in a large clinical trial.

Genome change – evolution and design

Our species, *Homo sapiens*, is only about half a million years old. Compare this to the 'living fossils', the Coelacanth, a fish largely unchanged for 400 million years, and the Ginkgo, a tree largely unchanged for 170 million years. Humans and mice diverged 60 million years ago. Population genetics define our genomic patterns, predict the causes of diseases and have implications for therapy.

Evolution – chance and selection

Natural selection is a driving force of evolution, wherein the most 'fit' animals survive to reproduce. Selection acts on the larger population of offspring that each generation produces. Absent selection, populations would increase geometrically at the rate determined by their fecundity. The agents of selection include predators, parasites and limiting factors, most often food. The individual offspring that are best adapted to the combination of stresses encountered by their generation are most likely to survive and reproduce. By defining fitness as survival, the dictum 'survival of the fittest' is rendered a (useful) tautology.

Selection does not operate directly on the genotype. Phenotype, not genotype, is what matters to the survival of an organism. In a simple genetic system, only homozygous recessive (*aa*) genotypes are apparent; the others (*AA* + *Aa*) look the same. Fortunately, we can calculate the allele frequency from the *aa* population alone. For example, if the frequency of the *a* allele is 1 in 20 (0.05 or 5%), then the frequency of *aa* genotypes is 1 in 400 (0.25%). Note that these calculations are based on probability alone, requiring no additional information about the population.

Hardy–Weinberg equilibrium – bad genes hide

Genotype frequencies were first rigorously calculated in collaboration between an English mathematician and a German physician. The Hardy–Weinberg equilibrium equation defines the relationship between the frequency of dominant and recessive alleles, symbolized here as *A* and *a*: $AA + 2 \times Aa + aa = A^2 + 2 \times Aa + a^2 = 1$. The frequency of the dominant allele can be observed because all of the homozygous (*AA*) and heterozygous (*Aa*) individuals display the trait. For example, if 75% of the population displays the phenotype of the dominant allele, then homozygous recessives are 25% ($a^2 = 0.25$) and the frequency of the recessive allele is 50% ($a = 0.5$). Therefore, the allelic frequency of A is also 50%. Now consider the case of a recessive allele present at 1% ($a = 0.01$). Although

~2% of the population would be heterozygous carriers, only 1 in ten thousand ($a^2 = 0.0001$) would be homozygous recessive individuals. Even if the recessive allele were deleterious, or even lethal, in a homozygote, only a small fraction would be selected against in each generation. This simple example illustrates the persistence of deleterious alleles.

Comparative genomics and model organisms

The genomes of many different organisms have been sequenced (Table 2.6). They range in size by a factor of two-hundred-million. The number of genes contained within the larger genomes is only an informed guess because of the difficulty in clearly identifying a gene. However, several families of genes can be identified in many different organisms. For example, several well described signalling pathways are conserved in flies and vertebrates, including several receptor tyrosine kinase pathways. Many components of these pathways are also found in the worm *Caenorhabditis elegans*.

Genome size does not correlate with complexity of the organism. The human genome is about 200 times larger than baker's yeast (*S. cerevisiae*) but 200 times smaller than a protozoan, *Amoeba dubia*.

Completing the sequence of the human genome represents only one step, albeit a large one, towards understanding how cells and organisms work. The next challenge is to identify genes and control regions within the sequence and determine their function. These tasks will be aided by comparisons with simpler organisms that perform some of the same tasks. For example, the regulation of cell death was discovered in worms and is now key to developing more effective cancer therapies. The complete genomes of many human pathogens have been completed and have proven invaluable tools in the rational design of vaccines.

Mouse genome sequence

Mice have been intensively studied since the beginning of the twentieth century because they

Table 2.6 Genome size correlates poorly with organism complexity or number of genes.

Organism	Form	Genome (Mb)	Cells	Genes
pUC19	Synthetic	0.003	(1)	2
SV40	Primate virus	0.01	(1)	5
M13	Bacteriophage	0.01	(1)	10
λ	Bacteriophage	0.05	(1)	66
Mycobacterium pneumoniae	Mycobacterium	0.82	(1)	677
Mycobacterium tuberculosis	Mycobacterium	4.4	(1)	3918
Escherichia coli	Bacterium	5	1	4289
Saccharomyces cerevisiae	Yeast	12	1	6200
Caenorhabditis elegans	Worm*	97	1000	18 400
Drosophila melanogaster	Fruit fly*	180	10 000	13 600
Homo sapiens	Mammal*	3100	>1 000 000 000 000	~23 000
Amoeba dubia	Protozoan	670 000	1+	?

*Haploid sizes are listed (most somatic cells have twice as much DNA). Genome size in millions of base pairs (Mbp). pUC19 is a synthetic cloning plasmid. Simian virus 40 (SV40) is a papovavirus that infects monkeys. Bacteriophages M13 and lambda (λ) are viruses that infect bacteria. Mycoplasm is an intracellular microbe. *M. pneumoniae* is one cause of pneumonia. *M. tuberculosis* causes tuberculosis. *E. coli* is a common laboratory and intestinal bacterium. *S. cerevisiae* is baker's yeast. The nematode *C. elegans* was the first multicellular organism whose genome was sequenced. The fruit fly *D. melanogaster* has provided important insights into gene function for a century. Mouse and human genomes are about the same size. Amoebas have life stages that are haploid and diploid, and unicellular and multicellular; this genome is not well characterized.

have proven to be invaluable aids in understanding human biology. Many mouse mutants display phenotypic similarities with human diseases. These animals permit insights into many human diseases, such as cancer, and normal processes such as development, immunity and ageing.

The public Mouse Genome Sequencing Project started in 1999 with the goal of sequencing the genome of the C57BL/6J inbred strain (abbreviated 'B6') by 2005. The Project integrates existing information about mutants and gene expression (www.informatics.jax.org/). The Celera company has sequenced four mouse strains, covering >99% of the mouse genome.

Transgenic animals – adding genes

Mice – key models of human disease

Some questions cannot be answered by studying cells in culture dishes. The ability to place new genes into animals has greatly advanced our understanding their function, especially those of genes involved in development or the immune system. Such technology may eventually allow the repair of disease-causing genes in humans.

Transgenic Animals

Transgenic animals have genes (transgenes) added to their genomes. The added genes can be from the same or a different species. This allows one to see the effect of *new*, *deleted* or *altered* genes (a gene is deleted when it is replaced by an inactive transgene).

The generation of transgenic mice followed the discovery that *embryonic stem* (ES) cells could be isolated from a blastocyst (an early developmental stage, around the time of implantation of the fertilized egg). ES cells could be grown *in vitro* and transfected with a gene (Chapter 1). When ES cells are mixed with fresh blastocyst cells and placed in a foster mother, they participate in the development of the mouse (Figure 2.18). The resulting mouse is a *chimera* (mix) of the original blastocyst cells and the ES cells grown *in vitro*. (A chimera originates

from more than one zygote; a mosaic animal develops from a single zygote.) In some chimeras, the germ tissues develop from the ES cells. These animals pass on the transgene to their progeny.

Adding DNA to Cells

Techniques for transferring DNA into eukaryotic cells are called *transfection*, from a combination of transfer and infection. These methods include precipitation, electroporation (shock) and lipid encapsulation. When viruses are manipulated to contain and transfer genes, the technique is called *transduction*. The modified virus is called a *vector*.

There are two types of transgenes.

1 *Random*: transgenes insert the genome anywhere. Multiple copies are usually found in the transfected cell and chimera. Some of these transgenes may come under the control of different gene promoters and be inappropriately regulated (Figure 2.19).

2 *Targeted* (*site-specific* or *homologous recombination*): the transgene *replaces* the original gene in the correct position in the genome. The frequency of homologous recombination is greatly increased by adding flanking DNA sequences that match the target region (Figure 2.20). Nonetheless, these transgenes can also insert randomly, so the cells containing only the correctly targeted genes must be selected.

Random transgenics are much easier to generate than are targeted transgenics. The principal difficulty with random transgenes is the inappropriate influence of unusual genetic neighbours. This can be evaluated by analysing several independently generated transfectants (cells that express the transgene product). Each independent transfectant is likely to have the transgene inserted into a different site in the genome, so the effects of different neighbouring genes are averaged out.

Transgenes have to date produced more sickness than health, which tells us something about the fragility of health. In transgenic mice, for example, overexpression of the normal cellular *myc* oncogene leads to adenocarcinomas, and expression of the viral SV40 transforming genes produces tumours.

Figure 2.18 Transgenic animals – making an animal out of cultured cells. (1) Embryonal stem (ES) cells are isolated from a blastocyst, which is removed from a pregnant female. (2) ES cells are grown in culture, where they are transfected with a transgene and stable transfectants are selected. (3) Transfected ES cells are injected into a second blastocyst, which is implanted into a foster mother. (4) Chimeric offspring are screened for germline transmission. The foster mother contributes no genes to the chimera. One formidable technical constraint has been that the ES cells can only be cultured for a limited time *in vitro* before they lose their ability to participate in the development of the animal. In some mouse strains, transgenics can be generated by adding DNA directly to the blastocyst.

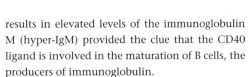

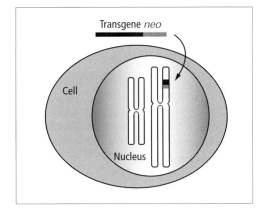

Figure 2.19 In preparation for making a transgenic animal, new genes called transgenes are inserted into the chromosomes of ES cells. ES cells are transfected with a gene of interest that is linked to a resistance gene. The drug resistance gene (here, the *neo* gene that confers resistance to the antibiotic neomycin) allows selection of the stable transfectants. These insert into the genome randomly. Selected ES cells are then infected into a blastocyst, which is implanted in a foster mother.

Deleting and adding genes: knockouts and knock-ins

Historically, natural mutations that reduce or eliminate the activity of the encoded protein have provided the first indication of the protein's function. For example, the immune deficiency that

results in elevated levels of the immunoglobulin M (hyper-IgM) provided the clue that the CD40 ligand is involved in the maturation of B cells, the producers of immunoglobulin.

> **Gene Knockouts**
>
> In 'knockout' animals, a gene is replaced with a mutant gene that does not encode the normal gene product.

Gene 'knockout' technology can provide exactly the mutant you want now, without waiting for an 'experiment of nature'. Knockout mice have already helped to define the function (or often the apparent dispensability) of many genes. Knockout mice are a subset of *targeted transgenes*, inserted by homologous recombination, in which the replacement gene is deleted or interrupted (Figure 2.20).

Remarkable genetic redundancy has been observed in many experimental systems, where the deletion of one gene has little or no apparent effect (phenotype). This can be a huge surprise, as when myoglobin knockout mice proved to be relatively normal. At the other extreme, some knockouts die as embryos because the deleted gene has an unexpectedly important role in development. The most illuminating knockouts have been those in which the deleted gene is important enough to cause a problem when it is missing and the

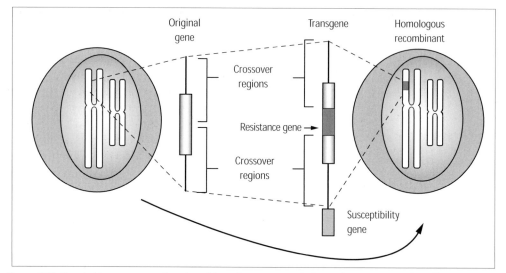

Figure 2.20 Targeted transgenes can 'knock out' homologous genes. A drug resistance gene and a different drug susceptibility gene are parts of the 'targeting construct', a large DNA that is used to knock out the endogenous gene. The resistance gene interrupts the gene that is targeted, resulting in a specific mutation of that gene. Large flanking regions encourage site-specific insertion by homologous recombination, which results in the loss of the susceptibility gene. The selected ES cells are then injected into a blastocyst. Although only one of the two genes in the cell is mutated, mating the heterozygous offspring could breed a homozygous mouse.

function can be inferred from the nature of the defect.

A gene's function can be refined by replacing the defective gene with a variant gene, a natural or designer allele. These are called 'knock-ins'. For example, the wild-type allele could be replaced with a suspected disease-causing allele.

Cloning animals – therapeutic cloning

Stem cells are cells that are able to regenerate themselves and, under certain conditions, develop into differentiated cell populations. The ultimate stem cell is the fertilized egg, which develops into all the different cells, tissues and organs of an entire animal and the germ cells for the subsequent generation. Commitment to cell fate is gradual. Cells of the zygote are *totipotent*, able to generate an entire animal. Cells from later in development are *pluripotent*, able to generate cellular subsets or tissues, such as haematopoietic cell lineages or leukocyte lineages.

Animals have been cloned by *somatic cell nuclear transfer*, where the nucleus of an ovulated egg is removed and replaced by a nucleus removed from an adult cell (Figure 2.21). In theory, cloning could be used to produce more animals with desirable characteristics. However, very few nuclear transfers lead to viable animals and these often suffer 'large animal syndrome' and other problems suggesting subtle developmental defects. More must be learned about the genome imprinting and other processes in natural development. The United Nations approved in 2005 a non-legally binding prohibition on all types of human cloning, despite calls to allow member states to make their own decisions regarding therapeutic cloning.

Therapeutic cloning envisions growing tissues and even organs for use in humans. Cloning should produce tissues indistinguishable from graft recipient's cells, thereby avoiding immune-mediated rejection, which is the key problem in current transplant regimens. Alternatively, it may be possible to coax cells from the patient to adopt stem cell properties. If we can identify the gene products that make the environment of the fertilized egg unique, it may be possible to add them to somatic cells and confer new regenerative properties.

Ethical, legal and social implications

There is hope, fascination and fear in molecular genetics. New biomedical technologies raise old and new ethical, legal and social implications (ELSI) questions.

• Humans could probably be cloned by adapting those techniques that are successful in other animals. Should it be permitted? If not, how should society prevent or discourage cloning? If so, can a clone donate organs to the original? Can a clone be developmentally manipulated? Some possibilities are ghoulish but might seem acceptable in certain cases. Human cloning has been banned in many countries.

• Xenotransplantation is the transplantation of tissues from non-human animals to humans. Transgenic pigs have been created to reduce immune rejection. However, alterations in the donor to promote graft success probably also reduce the natural barriers to pathogen exchange. For example, endogenous viruses from the donor species may easily infect the immunosuppressed human recipient. A retrovirus proliferating in a patient would be 'humanized' and thus pose a danger to all humans. A moratorium on xenotransplantation has been called for until the risks are better understood.

• Embryo selection can ensure that healthy children are born to high-risk parents, for example who are carriers for genetic disease. Few object when the alternative could be a child doomed to a short and miserable life. However, the ability to select genomes, and eventually to manipulate them, also raises the possibility of selection based on other traits, such as sex or appearance. Is it ethical to choose between embryos based on sex, appearance or intellect?

• Transgenic humans could probably be generated by inserting genes into *germ* cells. (Gene therapy usually envisions treating somatic cells.) Few would object to correcting mutations that cause human disease. Altering 'normal' genomes, however, might raise questions. For example, is it ethical to try to create people who are more athletic, intelligent or considerate?

• Embryonal stem cells are capable of differentiating into all tissues. Embryonal stem cells are unquestionably valuable in research and they are thought to have therapeutic potential. The assisted

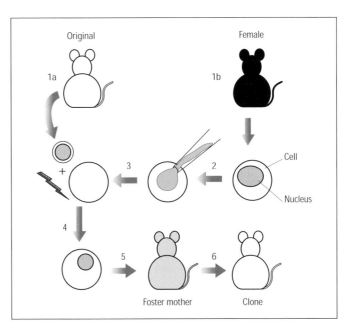

Figure 2.21 Animals are cloned by replacing an egg nucleus with a diploid nucleus from the original. A somatic cell is obtained from the original (1a) and an egg is obtained from a female donor (1b). The nucleus is removed from the egg (step 2–3), which is fused to the somatic cell by electric shock (4). In culture, the single cell embryo grows into the blastocyst. The blastocyst is transferred to a foster mother (5), which gives birth to the clone (6).

reproduction technology *in vitro* fertilization results in 'surplus' embryos, many of which are discarded, from which stem cells could be obtained. Is this, as some people believe, tantamount to murder? Research on new embryonal stem cells cannot receive federal support in the United States.

• Adult stem cells are not totipotent and they may not proliferate indefinitely. Nevertheless, they have been shown to differentiate into a wide variety of tissues. Moreover, they have the advantage of being derived from the patient, reducing infection risk and obviating immune tolerance problems. No substantive ethical questions have been raised regarding the use of adult stem cells.

• Genome sequence information will almost certainly help anticipate disease onset. Should this information be used for insurance pricing? Should it be available to employers? Will workers compete by *offering* their sequence information to potential employers?

• Human genes are already expressed in non-human organisms to make therapeutic molecules. Chimpanzees, close cousins of man, can be owned. What if chimp genes were systematically replaced with human genes? How many human genes make an organism 'too human'?

• Genome information will be invaluable for guiding medical care. However, genome information may be used for less noble purposes. For example, could an insurance company deny coverage to someone who possesses a disease-related haplotype?

Some of these questions may be resolved as the technologies are better understood. For example, recombinant DNA technology was once feared but is now widely regarded as relatively safe. Guidelines for safe recombinant DNA use are now incorporated into standard laboratory practices. Technical advances may moot some ethical questions. For example, embryonal stem cells lose their advantage if the growth and differentiation potential of adult stem cells can be increased.

To connect genetics and ethics on a different level, consider how traits like ethical behaviours evolve. An 'altruism gene' might increase the survival of genetically similar organisms. For example, since siblings share on average 50% of their genes, a sibling with low odds of mating could increase the odds of transmitting their own genes to the next generation by helping their nieces or nephews. Such behaviours are often observed in non-human animals.

Chapter 3

Genetics in clinical practice

An explosion in the number of diseases now recognized as being caused at least in part by genetic mutations directly results from the powerful and varied genetic technologies discussed in the preceding chapters. For instance, the number of genetic diseases and loci catalogued in Mendelian Inheritance in Man has risen from ~1500 in 1964 to >15 000 today. Since 1995, this catalogue has been available as Online Mendelian Inheritance in Man (OMIM) at http://www.ncbi.nlm.nih.gov/entrez/query.fcgi?db=OMIM. This chapter will present selected diseases currently known or thought to be genetically determined, and will highlight some of the genetic technologies that can assist in their diagnosis and/or treatment.

Genetic diseases

Inherited diseases result from a wide spectrum of genetic abnormalities, ranging from a single base change within a gene (as in sickle cell anaemia) to the loss or addition of a complete chromosome (as in Down syndrome). However, the most common human genetic diseases are polygenic resulting from the combined effects of multiple mutations, or genetic variations, at different loci, each of which has a small but additive effect. Onset or expression of disease also can be influenced by environmental factors, in which case the cause is said to be multifactorial.

Chromosome abnormalities

Description

Many chromosome abnormalities involve the loss or gain of entire chromosomes, as in Turner syndrome (Figure 3.1) and Down syndrome (Figure 3.2), or of changes in chromosome segments, such as duplications, deletions, inversions and translocations (*see* Chapter 2, p 60). Medical and developmental problems occur in these disorders as a result of gain, loss and/or disruption of one or more important genes. Human chromosome abnormalities are common occurring in ~1/2 of early miscarriages and 1 in 200 livebirths; their study can often aid in localization of disease-causing genes and provide insight into the pathogenesis of diseases in chromosomally normal persons in the general population. Specific examples of several common chromosome abnormalities are provided below.

Turner and Down Syndrome

In Turner syndrome only one intact X chromosome is present; all or part of the second X is deleted. This chromosome abnormality is common at conception and up to 15% of foetuses that spontaneously miscarry have Turner syndrome. Short stature and premature ovarian failure are cardinal features. Patients with Down syndrome have an extra chromosome 21. Characteristic features include typical facial appearance, congenital heart disease and mental retardation.

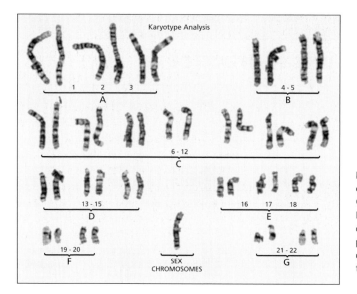

Figure 3.1 Karyotype of Turner syndrome (45, X). Karyotypes courtesy of Genetics Laboratories, Addenbrooke's Hospital, Cambridge. Chromosomes can be precisely identified by banding patterns. In addition, chromosomes can be assorted into seven groups (A to G) according to size and shape.

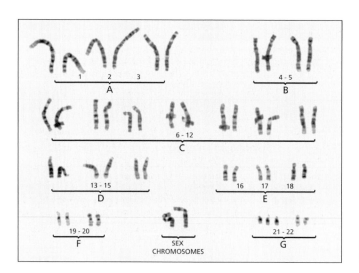

Figure 3.2 Karyotype of Down Syndrome (trisomy 21).

Diagnosis

Abnormalities that are greater than 5 million base pairs (Mbp) in size can routinely be detected by standard chromosome banding techniques. Increasingly, molecular cytogenetic techniques, such as fluorescent *in situ* hybridization (FISH, p 64; *see* Box, "Subtelomeric FISH", p 89) and comparative genomic hybridization (CGH, p 64) are used to detect smaller cytogenetic aberrations. FISH can detect 'microdeletion' syndromes, disorders caused by loss of a DNA fragment <5 Mbp in length. Microdeletions arise due to highly repetitive DNA, so-called duplicons (*See* Box, "Duplicons", p 89), that flank the commonly deleted segment and predispose to chromosome misalignment during cell division.

Duplicons

Low copy repeat DNA sequences found throughout the genome. The specific DNA sequence of duplicons varies according to chromosome region. Duplicons promote chromosome rearrangements by homologous recombination increasing the likelihood that the intervening sequence will be deleted, resulting in a microdeletion syndrome.

Subtelomeric FISH

Subtelomeric FISH analysis is able to detect minute alterations near the tips of human chromosomes (telomeres) not visible using standard chromosome banding. FISH screening of subtelomeric regions has resulted in the identification of previously unrecognized microdeletions and microduplications that cause mental retardation with and without additional congenital malformations.

FISH increases the diagnostic yield in cases with congenital malformations and/or mental retardation as well as guides the diagnosis and treatment of acquired chromosome abnormalities in selected malignancies (*see* Cancer section later in this chapter for details).

Treatment

Treatment for chromosome abnormalities by and large remains supportive. However, identification of genes altered in chromosome rearrangements has helped elucidate the genetic mechanisms underlying certain diseases in the general population.

Down syndrome

Clinical features

Down syndrome, most often caused by trisomy 21, affects ~1/1000 liveborns. A variety of medical problems are commonly found in persons with Down syndrome and include congenital heart disease, hearing loss, hypothyroidism, mental retardation and Alzheimer disease. Life expectancy has improved over recent decades with the current median age of death ~50 years of age.

Genes and Disease-related gene products

Over 300 genes map to chromosome 21 and three copies of certain critical genes, with subsequent overexpression of gene products, contribute to the Down syndrome phenotype. For example, it was proposed that early onset Alzheimer disease found commonly in Down syndrome was caused by having three copies of Amyloid beta Precursor Protein gene (*APP* located on chromosome 21q21). Amyloid accumulation is a neuropathological hallmark of Alzheimer disease. As persons with Down syndrome have three copies of the *APP* gene, it followed that they were likely to overproduce amyloid protein. This connection between genotype and phenotype identified *APP* as a candidate gene for Alzheimer disease; point mutations in *APP* were subsequently found in some kindreds in the general population with familial Alzheimer disease (*see* p 128).

Diagnosis

The diagnosis is typically confirmed using standard chromosome analysis; chromosome 21 interphase or metaphase FISH can also diagnose trisomy 21.

Treatment

Several medical management guidelines and screening protocols have been published which provide care standards and anticipatory guidance. Medication trials are underway in an attempt to prevent or minimize Alzheimer disease pathology.

Turner syndrome

Clinical features

Turner syndrome, caused by the partial or complete loss of an X chromosome in females, affects ~1/2500 liveborns. Its most common manifestations include short stature and premature ovarian failure, though additional medical problems, such as lymphatic abnormalities and congenital heart disease, can occur as well. Affected females generally have normal intelligence, but demonstrate a specific pattern of learning disabilities.

Genes and disease-related gene products

Over 1000 genes are located on the X chromosome, and loss of genes on Xp are critical for the Turner syndrome phenotype. Loss of the gene short stature homeobox (*SHOX*), located in the pseudoautosomal region at Xp22.33, appears to be responsible for the short stature found in Turner syndrome (*see* Box, "Homeobox", below). *SHOX* mutations in chromosomally normal individuals cause idiopathic short stature, as well as a relatively rare mild skeletal dysplasia (Leri–Weil syndrome) which has phenotypic overlap with Turner syndrome.

Diagnosis

Standard chromosome analysis establishes the diagnosis in most cases, but more than the usual number of metaphases should be analysed given the high frequency of X chromosome mosaicism; chromosome X interphase or metaphase FISH can also detect cases with loss of an entire X chromosome.

Treatment

Medical management and screening protocols have been published. Administration of growth hormone and oestrogen supplementation are considered standard of care, though details about dose and timing remain controversial.

Homeobox

A homeobox is a short stretch of DNA that encodes a 60 amino acid polypeptide whose sequence is virtually identical in all of the homeobox genes that contain it. Homeobox proteins containing this short polypeptide sequence are key regulators in embryonic development.

Williams–Beuren syndrome

Clinical features

Williams–Beuren syndrome, one of the best-recognized microdeletion syndromes, is caused by a ~1.5 million base pair deletion at chromosome 7q11.23. Cardinal features include vascular stenoses (narrowing or constriction of blood vessels), short stature, hypercalcaemia, mild mental retardation, and a characteristic intellectual and personality profile. The disorder almost always arises *de novo*.

Genes and disease-related gene products

Deletion of ~25 genes causes Williams–Beuren syndrome and several of these genes are proven to cause specific components of the phenotype. For example, numerous lines of evidence confirm that deletion of the gene elastin (*ELN*) causes the vascular stenoses of Williams–Beuren syndrome. This discovery paved the way to the finding that certain patterns of vascular stenoses in patients *without* Williams–Beuren syndrome were caused by *ELN* point mutations or intragenic deletions, proving that elastin protein haploinsuffiency (*see* Box, "Protein Haploinsufficiency", below) causes vascular stenoses.

Diagnosis

Since Williams–Beuren syndrome is a microdeletion disorder, the deletion is too small to be appreciated on standard chromosome analysis. FISH on metaphase chromosomes using a fluorescent elastin gene probe is the widely available diagnostic test of choice.

Treatment

Management and screening protocols have been published to provide guidelines for treating and/or preventing medical and personality problems.

Protein Haploinsufficiency

When dosage sensitivity of a gene product results in a phenotype. In other words, loss of one functioning copy of the gene leads to 50% of the protein product and produces a recognizable phenotype.

---

del 22q11 syndrome (diGeorge syndrome or Velocardiofacial syndrome)

Clinical features

This most common of the microdeletion syndromes, found in as many as 1/4000 persons, usually results from a ~3 Mbp deletion at chromosome 22q11. The same microdeletion underlies what had previously been considered two distinct entities, diGeorge syndrome and Velocardiofacial (VCF) syndrome.

In the developing embryo, neural crest cells, formed from the margin of the developing neural tube, migrate to many different locations and contribute to structures in the face, neck and chest. In del 22q11 syndrome disturbed neural crest cell migration causes a pattern of craniofacial, immunologic and cardiovascular anomalies which include facial dysmorphology, congenital heart disease [such as tetralogy of Fallot, or underdevelopment (hypoplasia) of the aortic arch], hypocalcaemia due to parathyroid gland underdevelopment, immune deficiencies and structural or functional abnormalities of the oral soft palate. Many patients have mild mental retardation and up to 25% go on to develop psychiatric problems, such as schizophrenia or depression.

> **Tetralogy of Fallot**
>
> Tetralogy of Fallot is a congential heart malformation consisting of four defects: a ventricular septal defect (hole between the two ventricles), obstruction to blood flow out of the right ventricle to the lungs, a right ventricle that enlarges to cope with the obstruction, and an aorta that is shifted to the right. It is often due to aberrant migration of neural crest cells into the heart during foetal development.

About 90% of cases are due to *de novo* deletions at 22q11, but the remaining cases are familial, sometimes with a previously undiagnosed parent transmitting the deletion to their offspring. Thus, del 22q11 syndrome acts as an autosomal dominant disorder, since an affected person has a 50 : 50 chance that each of their offspring will inherit the deletion.

Genes and disease-related gene products

The syndrome is produced by loss of about 30 genes from one chromosome 22q11, and it is the cumulative effect of missing several genes that appears to account for the phenotype. Loss of one copy of the gene *UFD1L* (coding for ubiquitin fusion degradation 1-like protein, which targets proteins for degradation by tagging an ubiquitin molecule onto them) or of *COMT* (catechol-O-methyl transferase, which codes for an enzyme that degrades catecholamines) could predispose to the psychiatric disease commonly seen in del 22q11 syndrome. Identification of the gene or genes responsible for the psychopathology found in del 22q11 patients could have important ramifications for the general population as mutations or variations in these same genes could contribute to mental illness in persons without a chromosome 22 deletion.

Diagnosis

Standard chromosome analysis detects a deletion or rearrangement involving 22q11 in <10% of patients with the disorder. The most reliable and accurate diagnostic test is FISH using a probe from the 22q11 critical region. This testing is widely available.

Progress towards therapy

Standard treatment involves providing care for existing medical and psychiatric problems and anticipatory guidance to prevent or minimize development of problems.

Single gene (Mendelian) disorder

Description

The genetic mutations responsible for thousands of single gene disorders are currently known. Disease-causing genes have been identified through various molecular techniques, such as cloning chromosome translocation breakpoints, linkage analysis, candidate gene analysis and identification of genes in model organisms. Now that the sequence of almost the entire genome is available through The Human

Genome Project, identification of mutations responsible for single gene disorders has become almost commonplace.

Diagnosis

Diagnostic techniques vary according to the type of mutation responsible for the disorder. Many point mutations are identifiable by PCR and sequencing. Diagnostic tests for single gene disorders are increasingly available through commercial laboratories which allow some common genetic tests to be ordered by the primary care physician. However, many single gene disorders such as Marfan syndrome or Ehlers Danlos syndrome continue to be clinically diagnosed because either the causative gene is unknown or is too complex for commercial testing. A careful physical examination and family history should always be completed when considering the diagnosis of a genetic disorder. The latter includes details on symptoms or diseases in relatives, parental consanguinity, recurrent miscarriages, mental retardation and birth defects.

Treatment

Treatment of single gene Mendelian disorders currently remains disease specific. Disorders due to mutations in structural proteins (such as Marfan syndrome or osteogenesis imperfecta) require supportive treatment designed to either prevent complications or to medically/surgically manage those that develop. Enzymatic disorders (such as inborn errors of metabolism like Phenylketonuria or Familial hypercholesterolaemia) can be successfully managed by selected dietary restrictions and/or medications that improve or bypass the enzymatic block. Recombinant technology has been instrumental in the development of enzyme replacement therapy which is the mainstay of treatment for certain enzyme deficiencies. Gene therapy of single gene disorders was initially heralded as the 'cure' for many genetic diseases but, unfortunately, it has achieved limited success, though it remains an area of great promise.

> **Gene Abbreviations**
>
> Abbreviations for gene names are written in italics. The *LDLR* (low density lipoprotein receptor) gene codes for a receptor protein of the same name, LDLR. Mutations in *LDLR* cause Familial Hypercholesterolaemia. In mice, only the first letter of a gene abbreviation is capitalized, for example, *Ldlr*. The human chromosome is indicated in parentheses, for example, *LDLR* (19p13).

Autosomal dominant disorders

Achondroplasia

Clinical features

Achondroplasia is the most common of the human skeletal disorders, affecting 1/20 000 to 1/40 000 livebirths. Individuals manifest short stature (with adult height of about 1.2 m) shortened limbs, exaggerated lumbar lordosis (swaybackness), and macrocephaly (enlarged head circumference) with frontal bossing (prominence). Medical problems include reduced muscle tone (hypotonia) in almost all infants along with an increased risk for cessation of breathing (apnoea) due to brainstem compression or obstruction of the airways. The most common complications during adulthood are obesity and compression of the spinal cord or spinal nerves due to narrowing of the spinal canal (spinal stenosis). Intelligence is usually normal. Over 80% of cases have no family history of achondroplasia and are caused by a *de novo* mutation on the paternally inherited chromosome #4, often in association with advanced paternal age.

Gene and disease-related gene product

Achondroplasia is always caused by a mutation in the Fibroblast growth factor receptor 3 gene (*FGFR3*) (4p16), which codes for a protein of the same name. Persons with achondroplasia are heterozygous for the *FGFR3* mutation. If two persons with achondroplasia have children, their offspring have a 1 in 4 chance of being *FGFR3* mutation homozygotes. This homozygosity produces a lethal short stature phenotype. The FGFR3 protein is a tyrosine kinase receptor that binds ligands belonging to the fibroblast growth factor family. Normally, ligand binding activates the receptor and initiates signal cascades important for cell growth and differentiation. The mutation responsible for achondroplasia causes constituitive (i.e. ligand-independent) activation of the FGFR3 receptor. Several different mutations in *FGFR3* result in skeletal dysplasias and the greater the extent of ligand-independent activation, the greater the severity of the dysplasia.

Diagnosis

The diagnosis is suggested by clinical findings and characteristic appearance on skeletal X-rays. Virtually all patients with achondroplasia have a mutation in the same *FGFR3* nucleotide (1138), suggesting this may be the most mutable nucleotide in the human genome. Mutation testing is clinically available.

Progress towards therapy

Current treatments include surgical correction of medical complications such as spinal stenosis. Options to maximize stature include growth hormone supplementation and/or surgical limb lengthening.

Adult polycystic kidney disease

Clinical features

The most common heritable renal disease, affecting 1/500–1/1000 persons, is an autosomal dominant condition in which renal failure results from progressive cystic degeneration of the kidneys. Cysts can also occur in other organs, including the liver; extra-renal anomalies such as vascular aneurysms, diverticular disease, hernias and cardiac valve abnormalities are more common in affected patients. Hypertension is often an early symptom.

Gene and disease-related gene product

Approximately 85% of cases are due to a defect in *PKD1* which maps to 16p13.3 and encodes the protein polycystin 1. The protein's exact functions remain unknown but it is a large membrane receptor, localized to renal epithelia cell cilia, that complexes with multiple proteins. Most mutations result in loss of function of polycystin. The *PKD2* gene, coding for polycystin 2, is responsible for most non-16p-linked polycystic kidney disease and has been localized to 4q13-23. Polycystin 2 is a voltage-activated calcium channel protein with structural homology to polycystin 1; it interacts with polycystin 1 and also localizes to the cilia of the renal epithelia. Patients with *PKD1* mutations have earlier onset disease and a more rapid progression to renal failure than patients with *PKD2* mutations.

Diagnosis

The diagnosis is strongly suggested by the characteristic appearance of renal cysts on sonography. Cysts increase in number over time. Almost 100 different mutations have been identified each in *PKD1* and *PKD2*. Commercially available testing is able to identify a mutation in 75% of patients with PKD1 and in an even higher percent of patients with PKD2. More than three-quarters of the *PKD1* gene is duplicated elsewhere on chromosome 16, so that screening for mutations requires care to ensure that they arise in *PKD1* rather than in the duplicated regions.

Progress towards therapy

Further characterization of the underlying functional defect should help to identify potential therapies. Approximately half of affected patients develop kidney failure by late middle age, requiring renal replacement therapy with dialysis or transplantation.

Charcot–Marie–Tooth, Types 1 and 2 (Hereditary motor and sensory neuropathies, HMSN)

Clinical features

Charcot–Marie–Tooth (CMT) disease, named for Drs Charcot, Marie and Tooth in 1886, refers to a group of neurologic disorders producing progressive muscle weakness and distal muscle atrophy, decreased deep tendon reflexes, distal loss of sensation and pes cavus (high arched foot). This very common group of neuromuscular disorders affects as many as 1/2500 persons. CMT, types 1 and 2, are both autosomal dominant disorders and symptoms generally develop between childhood and 30 years of age. There are numerous CMT subtypes, classified according to the speed of nerve conduction velocities, the mutant gene and the pattern of inheritance.

CMT1A is the most common subtype of CMT and is caused by a 1.5 Mbp duplication on chromosome 17p11. This results in duplication of the *PMP22* gene that codes for peripheral myelin protein 22. Nerve conduction velocity is slowed, as CMT1A is a demyelinating disorder. Ankle weakness with bilateral foot drop is very common, as an inverted 'champagne-bottle' appearance to the legs, due to lower leg muscle atrophy. Independent ambulation is generally maintained and life expectancy is normal.

CMT1B has a similar phenotype to 1A but is caused by mutations in the gene *MPZ* that codes for myelin protein zero.

CMT2 is clinically similar to the CMT1's, but generally has normal nerve conduction velocities and a milder phenotype. There are numerous CMT2 subtypes, and responsible mutations have been found in seven different genes.

Genes and disease-related gene products

CMT1A is a 'microduplication' disorder. Similar to the 'microdeletion' disorders discussed (*see* p 89), homologous stretches of DNA, or duplicons, flank the region and predispose to abnormal alignment and unequal crossing over of the chromosome 17's during meiosis. The critical gene in this duplicated region is *PMP22*. An extra copy of *PMP22* produces increased mRNA, which damages peripheral nerve myelin ultimately leading to axonal degeneration, by an unknown mechanism. Further increase in *PMP22* copy number, both in mice and humans, is associated with an increasingly severe phenotype. A small number of patients with CMT1A have a point mutation in *PMP22*, rather than duplication of the entire gene, resulting in a more serious phenotype. The highly deleterious effects of these mutations presumably occur through a 'dominant-negative' mechanism, whereby the mutant protein 'poisons' or eliminates normally functioning protein [*see* box "Dominant-negative Mutations", p 97]. Discussion of the mechanisms by which other genes cause CMT is beyond the scope of this book. Interestingly, while duplication of *PMP22* results in CMT, deletion of this gene causes a completely different disorder, hereditary neuropathy with liability to pressure palsies (HNPP). This is a peripheral neuropathy disorder associated with nerve palsies, such as peroneal palsy with subsequent foot drop, following minimal trauma.

Diagnosis

Nerve conduction studies should be the initial laboratory test when considering the diagnosis of CMT. Duplication of the *PMP22* gene responsible for CMT1A can be detected by FISH or Southern blotting; this testing is widely available. Very rarely, CMT is due to a point mutation in *PMP22*; gene sequencing to detect such mutations is also commercially available. Mutation testing in some of the other genes that cause CMT is available, in either a commercial or research laboratory. Additional genes responsible for CMT are likely to be identified in the future, as some families demonstrate linkage to chromosomal loci not yet known to house a CMT-causing gene.

Progress towards therapy

Treatment is supportive. Since many CMT subtypes follow an autosomal dominant pattern of inheritance, clinical and genetic examination of the first degree relatives of an affected individual is indicated. Animal models with *PMP22* mutations or extra copies of the entire *PMP22* gene demonstrate a demyelinating disorder comparable to human CMT; these models may identify the basis of the demyelinating process. Treatment with neurotrophic factors to prevent axonal death is an eventual possibility.

Familial Hypercholesterolaemia

Clinical features

Familial hypercholesterolaemia is the most common single gene disorder affecting lipid metabolism. It is usually caused by a mutation in the gene *LDLR* coding for the low density lipoprotein receptor protein. Approximately 1/500 persons are familial hypercholesterolaemia heterozygotes, carrying one mutant copy of the gene; these gene carriers have elevated low density lipoprotein (LDL) cholesterol levels with an increased risk for premature coronary artery disease. About 1/million persons are Familial hypercholesterolaemia homozygotes and have markedly elevated LDL levels and develop refractory atherosclerosis starting in childhood. This disorder follows a co-dominant pattern of inheritance: two copies of the mutant gene produce a more severe phenotype than a single copy.

Gene and disease-related gene product

Since free cholesterol is insoluble in water, it is transported in the blood attached to a carrier. Most cholesterol is delivered to the tissues for membrane and steroid hormone biosynthesis as part of a complex known as LDL, and this circulating LDL is removed by binding to the LDL receptor using a process known as receptor-mediated endocytosis. Defects in LDL receptor lead to elevated blood levels of LDL which promotes the development of atherosclerosis. The receptor is a transmembrane protein with several different functional motifs that aid in the binding of LDL particles. To date, many hundred different mutations have been identified in the *LDLR* gene (19p13), all of which result in the absence or diminution of receptor function (e.g. loss of receptor synthesis, loss of normal transport of receptor to the cell surface etc.).

Diagnosis

Diagnosis is generally based on family history, cholesterol history, presence or absence of xanthomas and results of a fasting lipid profile. Total cholesterol levels between ~9 and 13 mmol/l and between ~18 and 31 mmol/l are consistent with heterozygous and homozygous familial hypercholesterolemia, respectively; LDL cholesterol levels are the most significantly elevated. Since there are many different *LDLR* mutations, most unique to a given family, molecular methods are rarely used to establish the diagnosis in clinical practice.

Treatment

Homozygotes respond poorly to standard treatments but do show improvement following liver transplantation. Cholesterol levels can be lowered in heterozygotes by use of HMG CoA reductase inhibitors (so-called statins) and/or resins which prevent dietary cholesterol absorption from the gastrointestinal tract. Gene therapies, such as the introduction of a functioning *LDLR* gene, are currently being developed.

Hereditary Haemorrhagic Telangiectasia

Clinical features

Hereditary Haemorrhagic Telangiectasia (HHT), also known as Osler–Weber–Rendu syndrome, is a disorder of abnormal blood vessel formation whose features develop over time. The prevalence is estimated to be 1/10 000. Universal signs, present in all affected persons by age 40, are skin and mucosal telangiectasias (small arteriovenous malformations involving a direct connection between arteries and veins). Telangiectasias predispose to recurrent nosebleeds (usually present in childhood) and gastrointestinal bleeds. A substantial number of patients also suffer from large arteriovenous malformations, most commonly found in the lung, liver and brain. The lung vascular malformations can produce exercise intolerance and cyanosis due to abnormal admixture of arterial and venous circulations, but also can declare themselves by causing a pulmonary haemorrhage, a cerebral abscess or stroke. The brain vascular malformations produce non-specific symptoms such as headache and transient ischemic attacks, but stroke and haemorrhage may result as well.

Gene and disease-related gene product

Mutations in two genes cause HHT. Most cases of HHT are due to mutations in the gene endoglin (*ENG*, 9q34.1). These mutations lead to production of an abnormally truncated protein product, so that the features of HHT are caused by insufficient amounts of endoglin protein, so-called protein haploinsufficiency (*see* Box, "Protein Haploinsufficiency", p 88). The endoglin knockout mouse recapitulates the human phenotype. Endoglin is a membrane protein found on vascular endothelium, where it binds transforming growth factor-beta (TGF-β). It has been speculated that endoglin deficiency interferes with TGF-β's signalling on endothelial cells which, by an unknown mechanism, contributes to the blood vessel pathology of HHT. Mutations in a second gene, an activin A receptor, (*ACVRL1*, 12q11–14) cause ~20% of HHT cases. Its protein product is homologous to TGF-β; its precise mechanism of action in producing HHT also remains unclear.

Diagnosis

Clinical diagnosis is established when three of the following findings are present: telangiectasias, recurrent nosebleeds, positive family history or arteriovenous malformations. Genetic testing to detect *ENG* and *ACVRL1* mutations is clinically available. Mutations can be identified by sequencing the coding regions of the gene; quantitative PCR can supplement sequencing to detect deletions, rather than point mutations.

Progress towards therapy

Recurrent bleeds may require iron supplementation or even transfusions. The abnormal connection between a pulmonary artery and vein can be closed by transcatheter embolization, done in specialized centres. Knockout animal models of HHT may lead to a better understanding of the disease pathophysiology and eventually provide therapeutic insights.

Marfan syndrome

Clinical features

Marfan syndrome is a disorder affecting ~1/5000 individuals. Common musculoskeletal abnormalities include relatively tall stature with disproportionately long limbs and digits (compared to non-affected family members), scoliosis (curvature of the spine) and deformities of the sternum (pectus). Involvement of the cardiovascular system can be relatively minor (mitral valve prolapse in which floppiness of the mitral valve in the heart prevents normal closure) or life-threatening (dilatation of the aortic root, aneurysms [a weakness in the wall of a blood vessel causing abnormal widening], and/or dissection [a tear leading to separation of the layers of a blood vessel]). A variety of eye disorders, ranging from myopia to dislocation of the lens, are common. About 75% of cases are inherited from an affected parent, while the remaining 25% are *de novo*, that is, caused by a new mutation.

Gene and disease-related gene product

The *FBN1* gene (15q21.1) encodes fibrillin 1, a major protein component of microfibrils. Microfibrils determine the architecture of the extracellular matrix in connective tissue. A variety of missense and nonsense mutations in *FBN1* produce the Marfan phenotype. Fibrillin deficiency in a knockout Marfan mouse model leads to excessive activation of transforming growth factor-beta (TGF-β). TGF-β, a polypeptide hormone that typically functions in immune protection, regulates the production of connective tissue protein and its excess could contribute to some of the physical findings of Marfan syndrome.

Diagnosis

The diagnosis of Marfan syndrome is based on clinical consensus criteria established by a panel of experts, rather than a laboratory test. Findings from detailed physical examination, family history, slit-lamp ophthalmologic examination and an echocardiogram are combined to decide whether or not a patient has Marfan syndrome. Even though several hundred different mutations in *FBN1* have been identified, mutation screening is complicated and not routinely employed for diagnostic purposes. A fibrillin mutation is not always identified in persons clinically diagnosed with Marfan syndrome, and even among those in whom a mutation is found, it provides little prognostic information about the phenotype. In some families with confirmed *FBN1* mutations, the only clinical manifestations are aortic dissection or lens dislocation, giving rise to the concept of the 'fibrillinopathies', a spectrum of disorders due to mutations in the *FBN1* gene

Progress towards therapy

Current therapies are directed at preventing or treating medical problems, such as use of a beta-blocker antihypertensive agent to slow the rate of aortic root dilatation, or surgical repair of an already dilated aortic root. Frequent medical monitoring should include formal ophthalmologic examinations, echocardiography and scanning of major blood vessels to identify cardiovascular complications and treat them early in their course.

Osteogenesis imperfecta

Clinical features

Osteogenesis imperfecta (OI) is a disorder of collagen, affecting 1/10 000–1/20 000 livebirths, and is referred to in lay terms as 'brittle bone' disease. The hallmark features of the disorder involve excess bone fragility associated with decreased bone density leading to frequent fractures and abnormal long bone contour (such as bowing of the femurs). There can be additional connective tissue manifestations, all due to the underlying collagen defect, including blue discolouration of the sclerae, dentinogenesis imperfecta (discoloured fragile teeth), late onset hearing loss, short stature, scoliosis and joint laxity. The range of severity is extremely broad and is captured by classifying patients with OI into types I–IV, using the so-called Silence classification criteria. At the mildest end of the spectrum, patients with type I OI are relatively normal and suffer from fractures only following some degree of trauma. At the severe end of the spectrum, infants with the

so-called Type II perinatal lethal OI die from multiple fractures at birth.

Gene and disease-related gene product

The body contains numerous collagen moieties but most OI is caused by abnormalities in the most abundant collagen, type 1. Normally formed mature type 1 collagen is made of three chains, two coded for by the collagen 1A1 (*COL1A1*) gene and one coded for by the collagen 1A2 (*COL1A2*) gene. The three chains are able to form a tightly wound triple helix, in part because every third amino acid in the chain is a glycine, the smallest amino acid. OI results when a mutation leads either to the substitution of a bulky amino acid for one of the glycine residues, or when a decreased amount of structurally normal collagen is produced. Over 100 different mutations have been found to cause OI. Most are of the first variety described above, acting as a 'dominant-negative' mutation, in which an abnormally synthesized collagen chain interferes with normal assembly of the triple helix (*see* Box, below).

Dominant-Negative Mutations

Mutations that inactivate a function are usually recessive. Rarely non-functional mutations can be dominant if the mutant protein is expressed and interferes with the action of the normal protein by competing with it or in some way interfering with its normal role. Dominant-negative mutations can be created in the laboratory and can be used in research to identify protein function.

Diagnosis

The diagnosis of OI is suspected on clinical grounds and/or family history. Radiographic findings, such as osteopenia and Wormian bones (multiple bone islands seen on skull X-ray) are highly suggestive of the disorder. Definitive diagnosis can be established in ~90% of cases either by demonstrating a mutation in the Collagen 1A1 or 1A2 gene, or by documenting abnormal electrophoretic mobility of, or quantity of, the type 1 procollagen protein. Both of these tests are available in specialized clinical laboratories. The differential diagnosis of the infant with multiple fractures includes other genetic bone or skeletal disorders, and child abuse; sometimes laboratory testing helps to distinguish among these.

Progress towards therapy

Current therapy involves avoidance of fractures and treatment of those that do occur. Recent studies show that bisphosphonates, most commonly used to treat osteoporosis in postmenopausal women, increases bone density and decrease fractures in patients with OI. HLA-matched bone marrow transplantation (p 116) has been tried in patients with OI. The donor marrow provides a source of osteoblasts, which can synthesize collagen type 1 normally; unfortunately, only a small number of donor osteoblasts engraft, so there seems to be limited benefit from this treatment. Antisense RNA (RNAi p 23), to suppress the synthesis of the mutant collagen chain, has been attempted in OI mouse models and in fibroblasts taken from a patient with OI; although successful in mice, synthesis of both the abnormal and normal collagen chains was suppressed in the human fibroblasts. Other therapies being developed include a combined approach involving selective silencing of the mutant gene with RNAi, coupled with introduction of a normal collagen gene. These genetically corrected cells would then be reintroduced back into the patient as an autologous transplant.

Otosclerosis

Clinical features

Otosclerosis is the most common form of adult hearing loss. Hearing loss generally begins before the thirtieth birthday and progressively worsens at a slow pace. The disorder is autosomal dominant with incomplete penetrance (p 108). Abnormal growth of endochondral bone in the middle ear results in stapes fixation producing conductive hearing loss. In a minority of patients, the bone growth also extends into the inner ear compromising the

VIIIth cranial nerve, so that these patients have combined conductive and sensorineural hearing loss. Hearing loss is bilateral in most patients, especially in women. Tinnitus and balance problems can develop as well. Histologic evidence of otosclerosis can be found in 10% of Caucasians, though only a small minority develop clinically significant hearing loss. Otosclerosis is rare in African Americans and Japanese persons.

Genes and disease-related gene products

The genes responsible for otosclerosis have not been identified to date. However, linkage analysis (p 79) applied to autosomal dominant kindreds with multiple affected family members has identified at least three different chromosomal loci (chromosomes 15q25-26, 7q34-36 and 6p22.3-21.3). Thus, otosclerosis demonstrates considerable genetic heterogeneity, as mutations in at least three different genes result in the phenotype.

Diagnosis

Standard hearing (audiologic) evaluation can demonstrate hearing loss. A definitive diagnosis of otosclerosis requires surgical visualization of the middle ear.

Progress towards therapy

Current therapy involves hearing aids and in some cases surgical release of stapes fixation. Identification of the genes responsible for otosclerosis will likely lead to a better understanding of the pathogenesis of the disease and possibly provide insights into treatment or even prevention.

Porphyrias

Clinical features

The porphyrias are a group of several distinct disorders, sharing in common a defect in the synthesis of the oxygen-binding haeme component of haemoglobin. They are a rare example of a dominantly inherited metabolic disorder. King George III likely had porphyria and it has been suggested that Vincent van Gogh suffered from one of the porphyrias as well. The word derives from the Greek 'porphyr' meaning purple and, as will be explained below, some patients have port-wine discolouration of their urine during acute attacks. Selected porphyrias are presented below since a complete discussion is beyond the scope of this text.

Porphyrins (consisting of four pyrrole rings) are intermediates in haeme synthesis, a multi-step process controlled by several different enzymes. Symptoms, or attacks, of porphyria develop when an enzyme deficiency leads to the accumulation of haeme precursors, either predominantly in the liver (so-called hepatic porphyrias) or in the blood cells (erythropoietic porphyrias). Another classification scheme divides the porphyrias into whether neurological symptoms (acute porphyrias) or skin manifestations (cutaneous porphyrias) predominate. Symptoms of acute porphyrias typically develop after puberty and consist of bouts of severe abdominal pain and vomiting, muscle weakness and even paralysis, cranial nerve palsies, constipation due to ileus (lack of intestinal motility), hypertension and fluctuating psychiatric disturbance (including apathy, agitation and psychosis). All the symptoms are caused by haeme precursor toxicity to the autonomic and peripheral nervous systems. Females are symptomatic more frequently than males. Death from paralysis of respiratory muscles is a possibility in untreated patients. In the most common erythropoietic porphyria, erythropoietic protoporphyria, the haeme precursor, protoporphyrin, accumulates in the skin and symptoms start in childhood with pain and swelling of the skin following sun exposure. There are no neurological symptoms, but protoporphyrin can accumulate in the liver and produce liver damage, so this disorder is sometimes called erythrohepatic porphyria.

Genes and disease-related gene products

The most accurate method of classifying the porphyrias is according to their gene mutation and/or resulting enzyme deficiency. The most common porphyria, acute intermittent porphyria (AIP), caused by mutations in the porphobilinogen deaminase (*PBGD*) gene (11q23.3), results in ~50% deficiency of the enzyme porphobilinogen deaminase in the haeme synthetic pathway. Although AIP is autosomal dominant in inheritance, three-quarters of individuals who carry a mutant copy of *PBGD* never become symptomatic because nongenetic factors are also required to trigger an attack. Erythropoietic protoporphyria is caused by mutations in *FECH* gene (18q21.3) that codes for the enzyme ferrochelatase, the final enzyme in haeme biosynthesis.

Diagnosis

Most of the porphyrias are autosomal dominant disorders caused by partial deficiency of the enzymes in the pathway for haeme synthesis. Since genetic conditions due to enzyme deficiencies are usually autosomal recessive disorders, the porphyrias seem to be a striking exception and it is likely that complete absence of a haeme biosynthetic enzyme would be incompatible with life. Given the intermittent and protean nature of symptoms, the acute porphyrias are difficult to diagnose. During a porphyria attack, massive amounts of haeme precursors accumulate and these are responsible for the symptoms of the disorders. In AIP, large quantities of δ-aminolaevulinic acid (ALA) and porphobilinogen are excreted from the liver, and porphobilinogen is excreted in the urine. Upon oxidation of the porphyrins in room air, the urine becomes discoloured to the naked eye. Over 200 mutations have been identified in *PBGD*, with the majority of families harbouring a private (e.g. unique) mutation. Deficiency of the enzyme porphobilinogen deaminase can be documented in red blood cells even when patients are healthy between acute attacks; however, only one-third of mutation carriers demonstrate increased urinary porphyrins between attacks. Sequencing of *PBGD* as well as determination of cellular porphobilinogen deaminase enzyme activity are available in specialized laboratories. Erythropoietic protoporphyria (i.e. erythrohepatic porphyria) is also an autosomal dominant condition. Numerous mutations have been identified in *FECH* (18q21.3) and, biochemically, patients demonstrate massive amounts of protoporphyrin in red blood cells, faeces and plasma.

Treatment

Most acute attacks are precipitated by exposure to medication, alcohol, infection or calorie restriction. The list of drugs to be avoided is lengthy and a common pathogenic mechanism may involve up-regulation of haeme synthesis. Non-specific treatment of acute attacks includes removal of any inciting agents, hydration, glucose, pain control and management of electrolyte or neurological problems. Specific treatments aim to suppress haeme synthesis by inhibiting the first enzyme, ALA, in the pathway. Erythropoietic protoporphyria is treated by avoidance of sun exposure and close monitoring to detect those at risk for liver damage. Liver accumulation of protoporphyrin can be reduced by administration of a cholic acid but once liver damage occurs liver transplantation is the treatment of choice. Medications, other than oestrogens, do not exacerbate symptoms in the cutaneous or non-acute porphyrias.

von Willebrand disease

Clinical features

von Willebrand disease is the most common inherited bleeding disorder; 1% of the population is affected as determined by abnormal coagulation tests. However, only a small percent of these patients present with clinical manifestations of a bleeding disorder because the diathesis is generally mild. The most common symptoms are easy bruising, recurrent nosebleeds, and menorrhagia (excessive bleeding with menstrual periods). However, disease severity can vary among affected family members and even in the same individual over time. Most patients have von Willebrand disease, type I, due to decreased amounts of von

Willebrand factor (*see* below), accompanied by decreased levels of Factor VIII.

Gene and disease-related gene product

von Willebrand disease is caused by mutations in *VWF* (12p13.3). This gene codes for von Willebrand factor, which is exclusively produced by endothelial cells and megakaryocytes. von Willebrand factor plays a role in two aspects of normal haemo-stasis: (a) it allows platelets to attach to damaged areas of arterial vessels to initiate formation of a platelet plug; and (b) it stabilizes Factor VIII by covalently complexing with it. The latter function prevents degradation of Factor VIII making it available to participate in the coagulation cascade at the site of vascular damage. In the most common form of the disease, von Willebrand type I, symptoms are generally mild and are due to decreased amounts of structurally normal von Willebrand factor (as well as decreased Factor VIII level); both are generally reduced to 5–30% of normal. Other types of von Willebrand disease are due to structural or functional abnormalities in the von Willebrand factor, so that it improperly binds Factor VIII or platelets. A rare severe autosomal recessive form of von Willebrand disease exists, in which affected individuals have extremely low levels of von Willebrand factor and Factor VIII. Their bleeding abnormalities are very similar to those of patients with Haemophilia (p 114). Some autosomal recessive cases result from having two heterozygous parents with von Willebrand disease and inheriting the mutant copy of the gene from each parent.

Diagnosis

Widely available tests of coagulation that assess function of clotting factors, such as prothrombin time (PT) and activated partial-thromboplastin time (PTT), can be normal in von Willebrand disease and are, therefore, not of diagnostic value. The specific laboratory test known as 'bleeding time' is always prolonged in von Willebrand disease (as opposed to Haemophilia A where it is normal). However, more precise diagnostic testing is now available, such as measuring the plasma von Willebrand factor protein (von Willebrand factor antigen), or activity (ristocetin cofactor activity). Mutation analysis in the *VWF* gene can be performed in selected DNA diagnostic laboratories; however, it is rarely used in clinical practice as most mutations responsible for von Willebrand disease, type I, are not identified.

Progress towards therapy

Medications, such as aspirin and ibuprofen, that have anti-platelet effect should not be taken by persons with von Willebrand disease. Standard treatments for those with clinically significant bleeding problems include DDAVP (desmopressin inhaled as a nasal spray) which results in rapid increase in Factor VIII and von Willebrand factor levels, Factor VIII concentrates (which normally also contain von Willebrand factor) and antifibrinolytic agents. Administration of interleukin-11 in dogs leads to elevations in von Willebrand factor and Factor VIII that last considerably longer than those seen following DDAVP use; human studies are now needed.

Autosomal recessive disorders

Adenosine deaminase deficiency

Clinical features

Adenosine deaminase (ADA) deficiency was the first identified cause of severe combined immune deficiency (SCID), and accounts for approximately 15% of all SCIDs. Patients have varying degrees of T- and B-cell dysfunction. Patients with SCID secondary to ADA deficiency present in infancy and usually suffer an early death. Milder, later onset forms develop less severe infections with gradual immunologic deterioration. Patients with 'partial' ADA deficiency have decreased enzyme activity in red blood cells, but show 5 to 80% of normal enzyme activity in leucocytes and other nucleated cells. Heterozygote carriers with only 10% of ADA activity can have normal immune function.

Gene and disease-related gene product

Adenosine deaminase (*ADA*, 20q12-13) catalyses the deamination of adenosine and deoxyadenosine. The gene product is widely expressed in body tissues, but ADA deficiency predominantly affects lymphocyte function, because the purine products deoxyadenosine (dAdo) and deoxyadenosine triphosphate (dATP) build up in lymphocytes, with profound effects on their development and function. About 70 known mutations, the majority missense, have been described. Certain mutations have been associated with milder phenotypes.

Diagnosis

The disorder is diagnosed by failure to detect adenosine deaminase enzyme activity in red blood cells or lymphocytes.

Progress towards therapy

Some patients respond to enzyme replacement therapy by intramuscular injection of ADA which has been conjugated with polyethylene glycol (PEG) to increase its half-life. Successful bone marrow transplantation cures the immunological defect, but HLA-mismatched transplants have poor survival outcomes. ADA-producing lymphoid cells appear to have a growth advantage in successfully transplanted ADA-deficient patients. Furthermore, full immune reconstitution has been observed even if only T lymphocytes from the donor engraft.

Several features made ADA deficiency suitable for the first human gene therapy trial:
- the gene for ADA was cloned in 1983 and is relatively small with a cDNA of about 1.1 kb;
- a functioning copy of the gene that corrects the immunological defect can be introduced into lymphocyte progenitors *in vitro*, and these corrected cells can then be infused back into the patient;
- partial restoration of enzyme activity was predicted to be sufficient to restore normal lymphocyte function.

In 1989 the National Institutes of Health (NIH) Recombinant DNA Advisory Committee (RAC) gave approval for the first trial. A 4-year-old and a 9-year-old girl who had not fully responded to treatment with ADA–PEG were enrolled in the trial in 1990. T lymphocytes were isolated from their peripheral blood, transduced with a modified retrovirus containing the functional *ADA* gene, propagated in culture and reinfused back into the girls. This procedure was repeated at approximately 2-monthly intervals for 2 years. Both children continued with enzyme replacement therapy. Peripheral blood T-lymphocyte counts increased in both children, and tests of cell-mediated and humoral immunity improved. The long-term clinical benefit of this first gene therapy trial have been difficult to evaluate because it is unclear how much of any immunological improvement could be attributed to gene correction, the infusion of *in vitro* expanded and activated T cells or continued enzyme replacement. However, 10 years after the last cell infusion, approximately 20% of the first patient's lymphocytes continued to express the retroviral gene. In contrast, no expression of the transgene was detectable in lymphocytes from the second patient who developed persisting antibodies to components of the gene transfer system.

A neonatal trial involved three patients in whom a prenatal diagnosis of ADA deficiency was made. CD34+ (CD stands for cluster of differentiation) bone marrow progenitor cells were harvested from umbilical cord blood, transduced with a modified retrovirus containing the functional *ADA* gene, and infused intravenously on the fourth day of life. Transduced leucocytes could be detected in peripheral blood and bone marrow for 18 months. However, the number of ADA-producing cells, and the level of circulating ADA activity, remained low, and all patients needed to continue on ADA–PEG replacement therapy.

There is some evidence that continued use of PEG–ADA during gene therapy may reduce the survival of genetically modified lymphocytes. In a more recent study successful gene therapy for ADA-deficient SCID was achieved in patients who had not received PEG–ADA, but received modified CD34+ cells in combination with treatment to suppress bone marrow activity. Sustained engraftment of the engineered haematopoietic stem cells with differentiation into multiple lineages resulted in increased lymphocyte counts and improved immune functions.

A similar approach has recently been successfully used to treat X-linked severe combined immunodeficiency (X-SCID), which is caused by mutations in the gamma subunit of the interleukin-2 receptor (*IL2RG*), resulting in disruption of development of T lymphocytes and natural killer cells. In a French trial, *IL2RG* was inserted into blood stem cells of patients with X-SCID using a vector derived from a defective Moloney murine leukaemia virus. However, three patients subsequently developed a leukaemia-like disease, probably due to insertion of the retroviral vector near the promoter for a proto-oncogene (*see* p 132) known as *LMO2* (*LIM domain only 2*, which plays a crucial role in bone marrow development), leading to uncontrolled clonal proliferation of T cells. This complication underscores one of the potential risks of gene therapy.

Alpha 1-antitrypsin deficiency

Clinical features

Alpha 1-antitrypsin (α1-antitrypsin) is the major serine-proteinase inhibitor present in blood whose main function is to inhibit the enzyme neutrophil elastase. (Serine-proteinases are a group of proteolytic enzymes, including trypsin, chymotrypsin and elastase, in which the amino acid serine forms part of the active enzyme site.) Deficiency of α1-antitrypsin predisposes individuals to liver disease and lung disease. Affected adults can develop emphysema and bronchiectasis. Environmental factors, such as smoking, accelerate the rate of lung disease. Liver disease can present as hepatitis or cholestasis during infancy. During adulthood, there may be subclinical hepatic involvement, or significant disease with cirrhosis, followed by an increased risk for hepatocellular carcinoma. The prevalence of α1-antitrypsin deficiency is highest in northern and western European countries, affecting as many as 1/1500 individuals. However, the disease is found in all ethnic groups and is probably underdiagnosed worldwide.

Gene and disease-related gene product

The gene (14q32) which codes for the α1-antitrypsin protein is known as protease-inhibitor 1, or *PI*. Normally, a protein referred to as the 'M' subtype is translated. The two most common mutations give rise to 'S' and 'Z' variants, in which abnormal folding of the protein alters both its structure (favouring formation of polymers which may become deposited in the endoplasmic reticulum of organs such as the liver) and function.

Diagnosis

The diagnosis of α1-antitrypsin deficiency is usually established by isoelectric focusing, which measures the mobility of the α1-antitrypsin protein. Normal protein migrates in the middle and is designated 'M'; abnormally fast migrating proteins are designated A-L, while abnormally slow ones are designated N-Z. The most common mutations results in abnormal proteins referred to as 'S' and 'Z'. Patients who are homozygous for the 'Z' allele have only ~10% of normal enzyme activity. Mutation analysis in the *PI* gene can be performed to confirm the diagnosis and this testing is clinically available. Z-Z homozygotes and S-Z compound heterozygotes are at risk for developing lung and liver disease, while S-S homozygotes remain asymptomatic.

Progress towards therapy

Avoidance of smoking is key to minimizing lung damage. Administration of pooled human α1-antitrypsin has a modest benefit in slowing the progression of lung disease; it is available in the United States but not in the United Kingdom. Population screening by use of isoelectric focusing has been advocated so that persons homozygous for the 'Z' protein can be identified pre-symptomatically and be told not to smoke; however, this remains controversial. Lung or liver transplantation has been performed in occasional cases. A normal copy of the α1-antitrypsin gene has been successfully inserted

in liver and muscle tissue in model organisms; no human gene therapy trials have been performed to date.

Congenital adrenal hyperplasia

Clinical features

Congenital adrenal hyperplasia (CAH) refers to a group of enzymatic blocks in the synthesis of cortisol by the cortex of the adrenal gland. The resulting decreased levels of cortisol signal the pituitary gland to secrete adrenocorticotropic hormone (ACTH), which stimulates the adrenal cortex; persistently elevated ACTH leads to excess synthesis of other steroid precursors and eventual hyperplasia of the adrenal gland. More than 90% of patients have CAH due to 21-hydroxylase deficiency blocking the conversion of 17-hydroxyprogesterone to 11-deoxycortisol. The disorder affects ~1/15 000 individuals; general population screening programmes demonstrate that 1 in 4 Hispanics, 1 in 5 Ashkenazi Jews and 1 in 10 Italians are asymptomatic carriers of a mutant gene. Classical congenital 21-hydroxylase deficiency is diagnosed in female infants due to virilization of female external genitalia (as the enzyme block results in increased adrenal androgen synthesis); internal female genitourinary tract development is normal. About 75% of affected male and female infants experience salt-wasting, often presenting with decreased concentrations of sodium and elevated potassium (due to impaired aldosterone synthesis); dehydration and shock can develop within the first month of life, a so-called salt-wasting 'crisis'. Females with non-classical or later-onset CAH are normal at birth but usually demonstrate signs of excess androgen starting in puberty, such as hirsutism, delayed or irregular menses, polycystic ovary disease or infertility; males with this form of CAH may be asymptomatic or present with premature virilization.

Gene and disease-related gene product

Mutations in the gene *CYP21A2* (6p23.1) cause both classical and non-classical 21-hydroxylase deficiency. The gene, which lies within the HLA complex on chromosome 6 (Box, "Human Leucocyte Antigens", p 127), codes for a cytochrome P450 protein which hydroxylates steroids at the 21 carbon-position, a step required for both cortisol and aldosterone synthesis. *CYP21A2* is physically near a highly homologous pseudogene, *CYP21A1*, which likely arose through gene duplication; other genes in this region are also duplicated. These gene duplications (resulting in stretches of highly homologous DNA) predispose the *CYP21A2* gene to undergo structural changes, such as deletion, duplication and gene conversion to the non-functioning pseudogene, *CYP21A1*.

Diagnosis

All persons with 21-hydroxylase deficiency have elevated 17-hydroxyprogesterone (17-OHP) concentrations; higher concentrations are found in patients with classical CAH, compared to those with non-classical CAH. Newborn screening programmes utilize this finding and measure 17-OHP on spots of blood taken from the heel of a newborn and dried onto filter paper. Two-thirds of the states in the United States mandate newborn screening for 21-hydroxylase deficiency. This early screening is done in an attempt to identify affected infants before onset of a salt-wasting crisis. Chromosome analysis, or FISH, to look for the X and Y chromosome is required as part of the diagnostic work-up of an infant with ambiguous genitalia. An ACTH stimulation test distinguishes classical from non-classical cases, but is not accurate for diagnosing phenotypically normal carriers (e.g. those who carry a single mutant gene). Genetic testing is widely available and can detect >80% of the common gene changes; sequencing is also available to identify rare mutations. Patients who are homozygous for severe mutations that eliminate all 21-hydroxylase activity have classical CAH; those who carry one severe mutation and one mild mutation or two mild mutations are likely to have non-classical CAH. Carriers are most accurately diagnosed by genetic testing.

Treatment

Treatment of classical CAH consists of glucocorticoid replacement and mineralocorticoid replacement, for those with salt-wasting. Surgical reduction of an enlarged clitoris and/or vaginoplasty in a virilized female is done in some centres, but there is controversy whether surgery is best done in infancy or adulthood. Non-classical CAH may not require treatment, but signs of excessive androgen production can be corrected with low dose steroids. Administration of dexamethasone to a pregnant woman whose female foetus is confirmed to have classical CAH diminishes virilization of the external genitalia. Newer treatments combining low-dose glucocorticoid replacement with androgen receptor antagonists and blockers of androgen to oestrogen conversion are underway. Curative treatment using gene therapy is being attempted in model organisms. Adrenal injection of an adenovirus transduced with *CYP21A2* in a CAH mouse resulted in expression of the human gene.

Cystic fibrosis (Disorders of CFTR)

Clinical features

Cystic fibrosis is the most common life-threatening autosomal recessive disorder in Caucasians, affecting 1 of 2500 newborns. The disease results from a defect in the cystic fibrosis transmembrane conductance regulator (CFTR), a cyclic AMP-regulated chloride transporter; the gene was identified in 1989 by positional cloning.

Mutations in the *CFTR* gene lead to impaired chloride secretion from epithelial cells of numerous organs, notably, the respiratory tract, and ducts of the male genital tract, liver and exocrine pancreas. Impaired chloride transport results in production of abnormally viscous secretions that, in classical cystic fibrosis, are associated with recurrent chest infections and subsequent pulmonary damage, as well as obstruction of pancreatic and biliary ducts. Median survival is now ~30 years with most morbidity and mortality still relating to pulmonary disease. A variety of phenotypes that are milder than classical cystic fibrosis, so-called CFTR-opathies, are also due to mutations in *CFTR*. The best characterized CFTR-opathy is congenital bilateral absence of the vas deferens (CABVD) associated with male infertility. Mild chronic sinopulmonary disease and idiopathic pancreatitis, can also be caused by *CFTR* mutations (*see* below).

Gene and disease-related gene product

CFTR (7q31.2) functions as a cAMP-regulated chloride channel on the apical surface of airway and other epithelial cells. The single most common mutant allele is a 3 bp deletion which results in the loss of phenylalanine at position 508 (the ΔF508 mutation) from the mature protein. This accounts for ~70% of mutant alleles in Caucasians with cystic fibrosis. The ΔF508 mutation prevents the CFTR protein from reaching its site of action on the apical cell membrane. The remaining mutations interfere with the synthesis, intracellular trafficking or function of the CFTR protein. Individuals with milder phenotypes usually carry one severe mutation and one milder mutation.

Diagnosis

Diagnosis of cystic fibrosis is based on the combination of suggestive clinical symptoms, elevated chloride levels on a standardized sweat test, family history and genetic testing to identify the presence of *CFTR* mutations. Over 1000 CFTR mutations have been identified to date; the frequency of specific mutations varies according to ethnic group, with the ΔF508 mutation being the most common in all ethnic groups. Mutation panels, using PCR to detect the most common mutations, are widely available in clinical DNA diagnostic laboratories. If this type of targeted mutation analysis does not identify a mutation, then full gene sequencing, which identifies ~99% of all *CFTR* mutations, can be performed in selected laboratories.

Progress towards therapy

Conventional therapy for cystic fibrosis is symptomatic; it includes the administration of pancreatic enzymes to aid in protein and fat absorption and intensive treatment of chest infections with physiotherapy and antibiotics. DNA released from necrotic inflammatory cells contributes to the viscosity of the sputum in cystic fibrosis. Recombinant human deoxyribonuclease (rhDNase) has been developed as a mucolytic agent, and although effective, it is expensive. Curative treatment is being attempted through gene therapy and several treatment trials using different vectors have been completed. The NIH gene therapy trial for cystic fibrosis was approved in 1992. A modified adenovirus containing the *CFTR* gene was delivered by bronchoscopy into the lungs of four adult patients; subsequently epithelial cell *CFTR* gene expression was demonstrated in all patients. However, the efficiency of transduction was low, and no patients had evidence of continued gene expression beyond 10 days after treatment. One patient who received the highest dose of adenoviral particles developed fever, hypoxia and pulmonary infiltrates which were attributed to an inflammatory reaction to the adenoviral vector. Other studies have demonstrated transient correction of the chloride transport defect through adenoviral-mediated transduction of the *CFTR* gene in nasal epithelium. Some patients suffered from localized inflammation, and the development of an immune response against the virus limits its effectiveness as a vector since repeated administration is necessary. Liposomal-mediated transfer of plasmid DNA containing the *CFTR* gene provided an alternative method of gene delivery which is well tolerated, but not efficacious as chloride transport is only briefly restored after plasmid delivery into nasal and lung epithelium. Attempts are underway to transfer a compacted *CFTR* gene directly into the airway.

Familial Mediterranean fever

Clinical features

Familial Mediterranean fever (FMF) is an inflammatory disorder with recurrent episodes of fever and pain that are caused by inflammation of the lining of the abdomen, heart or joints (leading to peritonitis, pericarditis or synovitis). These episodes can last several hours or even days. The abdomen is the most frequent site of pain, sometimes prompting a laparotomy. Amyloidosis can develop in untreated patients. FMF is most common in persons of Mediterranean descent, such as non-Ashkenazi Jews, Armenian Arabs and Turks. As many as 1 in 5 persons in these ethnic groups are gene carriers. FMF is not restricted to persons of Mediterranean heritage, though it is usually associated with milder mutations in other populations.

Gene and disease-related gene product

The familial Mediterranean fever gene, *MEFV* (16p13.3) is expressed in white blood cells. It encodes the protein marenostrin, also known as pyrin, containing protein motifs seen in the programmed cell death pathway. Pyrin is expressed predominantly in neutrophils and monocytes, and is thought to regulate inflammatory responses through activation of caspase-1 leading to both inflammation and apotosis (*see* Box, below). Mutations in pyrin lead to an exaggerated inflammatory response that results in the typical symptoms of an FMF attack.

Caspases and Apotosis

Caspases (cysteinyl aspartate-specific proteases) are enzymes that cleave specific proteins at aspartate amino acids. The first member of the caspase family was discovered in the nematode *C. elegans* and was termed Ced-3 (Cell Death-3), because mutations in the gene encoding Ced-3 prevented the programmed death of cells during development of the worm. Ced-3 was later found to be similar to the mammalian gene caspase-1. At least 14 caspase isoforms have now been identified. These isoforms play key roles in both inflammation and apotosis. Apotosis is a genetically programmed series of events leading to the death of a cell in which the cell fragments into membrane bound particles that are then engulfed by phagocytes or immune cells without eliciting an inflammatory response.

Diagnosis

Acute phase reactants are elevated during an attack and are suggestive of FMF. The diagnosis can be confirmed by commercially available *MEFV* mutation testing.

Progress towards therapy

Standard treatment remains daily colchicine. Further elucidation of the role of pyrin should improve understanding of FMF, and other inflammatory conditions, and help identify environmental triggers that can lead to attacks.

Gaucher disease, type 1

Clinical features

This form of Gaucher disease is a lysosomal storage disorder affecting as many as 1/500 persons of Ashkenazi Jewish descent, but also found in all ethnic groups, though at much lower frequencies. The sphingolipid, glucocerebroside, accumulates in the liver, spleen and bone marrow. Low white and red cell counts, thrombocytopenia, enlargement of the liver and spleen, and bone involvement ranging from osteopenia to osteonecrosis are common. Non-specific symptoms such as fatigue, bone pain and jaundice can also occur. Patients with type 1 Gaucher disease do not have involvement of the central nervous system.

Gene and disease-related gene product

The *GBA* gene codes for the enzyme glucocerebridase (also known as glucosylceramidase) (1q21), which metabolizes glucocerebroside. Over 200 mutations have been identified to date. Mutations responsible for type 1 Gaucher generally result in 10–15% of normal enzyme activity. Other mutations associated with more profound enzyme deficiency produce the neurologic problems seen in types 2 and 3 Gaucher disease.

Diagnosis

The diagnosis is suggested on bone marrow examination, following detection of 'Gaucher cells', macrophages filled with insoluble lipids. The diagnosis is confirmed by biochemical determination of glucocerebridase level in leukocytes. Molecular testing is widely available, especially for the four common mutations responsible for ~90% of Gaucher cases in Ashkenazi Jews. Unfortunately, genotype–phenotype predictions are limited; both inter-familial and intra-familial variability exist even among patients with the same mutation. Many persons homozygous for the N370S mutation never develop clinical symptoms. The inability to prognosticate the clinical course and natural history based on genotype limits the utility of population and prenatal screening for Gaucher disease. A highly homologous nearby pseudogene can interfere with molecular diagnosis of the disorder.

Progress towards therapy

In 1991, intravenous infusion of a modified form of the glucocerebridase enzyme that selectively targets macrophages became available as a form of enzyme replacement therapy. Although this treatment is well tolerated and is very effective for reducing hepatosplenomegaly and its accompanying symptoms, twice monthly infusions are needed and their annual cost can be as high as $100 000. Another form of therapy blocks the formation of glucocerebroside so that the patient's own residual enzyme activity is sufficient to prevent build-up of substrate. Curative treatment by retroviral-mediated transfer of the human glucocerebridase gene into CD34+ has been performed in a limited number of Gaucher patients, raising the prospect that retroviral transduced haematopoietic stem cells will ultimately provide gene therapy. However, sustained increase in glucocerebridase activity did not occur.

Haemoglobinopathies

Clinical features

Normal adult haemoglobin is made up of two polypeptide chains, the alpha- and beta- chains, which are folded such that each chain can hold an oxygen-binding haeme molecule. The haemoglobinopathies are a diverse group of autosomal recessive disorders of haemoglobin synthesis which include sickle cell anaemia (abnormal

beta-chain synthesis) and the thalassaemias (deficient or absent alpha- or beta- chain synthesis). Together they form the most common group of single gene disorders in the world population.

Genes and disease-related gene products

Genes encoding five different beta-globin chains and three different alpha-globin chains are expressed in a precisely regulated manner during different stages of development. For example, during foetal life beta-globin variants called gamma-globin combine with alpha-globin chains to give rise to foetal haemoglobin. During adult life the beta-globin proteins combine with alpha-globin chains to form adult haemoglobin. All five beta-globin chain genes are clustered on chromosome 11, whereas the alpha-globin chain genes occur together on chromosome 16. Numerous different mutations in the alpha-globin and beta-globin genes have been described, which give rise to alpha or beta thalassaemia, respectively. Sickle cell anaemia is caused by a point mutation, which involves substitution of T for A in the second nucleotide of the sixth codon, changing the sixth amino acid from glutamine to valine (*see* p 60).

Diagnosis

Haemoglobinopathies are diagnosed either by detection of mutant haemoglobin protein (using various detection techniques, such as liquid chromatography, isoelectric focusing or haemoglobin electrophoresis) or by genetic analysis, using mutation detection or gene sequencing.

Progress towards therapy

Treatments for severe thalassaemias include transfusions, chelation, splenectomy and/or bone marrow transplantation. In addition to the above treatments, patients with sickle disease can receive hydroxyurea to increase the production of foetal haemoglobin, which acts to stabilize the abnormal haemoglobin. These disorders are excellent targets for gene therapy. For example, transduction of a normally functioning globin gene into haematopoietic stem cells using lentivirus vectors has shown promise in animal models. Alternate strategies are also being explored in animal models, such as reactivation of silenced foetal or embryonic globin genes.

Hereditary haemochromatosis

Clinical features

Hereditary haemochromatosis is a common disorder leading to excess iron absorption and iron deposition, chiefly in the liver, pancreas, heart, synovial membranes and endocrine glands. Symptom onset generally begins during the fourth or fifth decade of adult life. Abnormalities can include cirrhosis, with an increased risk of developing hepatocellular carcinoma, diabetes mellitus, cardiomyopathy, arthropathy (joint damage) and hyperpigmentation ('bronzing') of the skin. In some patients, less severe symptoms, such as lethargy, arthralgia (joint pains) and impotence, are the only manifestations but, in fact, the majority of homozygotes do *not* manifest any clinical disease at all. Some experts believe the penetrance (*see* Box, below) of Hereditary haemochromatosis is <1%, but others believe it is as high as 10–20%, depending on the criteria used for diagnosis. In some northern European Caucasian populations, 12–15% of persons are heterozygous mutation carriers and about 1/150 persons are homozygous mutation carriers. Males are more commonly symptomatic than premenopausal females.

Penetrance

Penetrance describes the frequency with which phenotypic manifestation of a gene are expressed. A highly penetrant gene will express itself almost regardless of the effects of environment or other interacting genes, whereas a gene with low penetrance produces characteristic features much less often.

Gene and disease-related gene product

Mutations in the *HFE* gene are the most commonly identified cause of hereditary haemochromatosis. The *HFE* gene (6p21.3) codes for a protein that resembles major histocompatibility complex class I proteins and that is important for cellular iron transport. In symptomatic Caucasian patients, the single most common mutation in *HFE* is Cys282Tyr (C282Y) and the second most common is His63Asp (H63D). Together, they account for ~90% of the mutant alleles in patients with clinical evidence of disease.

Predicting disease risk based solely on genotype is challenging. C282Y homozygotes are the most likely to develop clinically significant disease with one-third showing evidence of iron overload and another one-third developing end-organ disease. Patients who are compound heterozygotes (C282Y/ H63D) have no more than a 2% risk of developing disease, while homozygous H63D mutation carriers have virtually no risk of clinical disease. Thus, most Caucasians who carry a common mutation in each of their HFE alleles never become symptomatic. In southern Europeans and in Africans, hereditary haemochromatosis has a variety of genetic causes, none of which is present in more than a few percent of individuals, unless there has been admixing with northern Europeans. Other factors such as alcohol consumption and genetic modifiers (e.g. the interacting effects of other, as of yet unknown genes) influence expression of the disorder.

Diagnosis

A combination of screening blood tests, particularly transferrin saturation and serum ferritin, are able to document the presence of iron overload. Mutations in the *HFE* gene can be detected in the majority of affected Northern European Caucasians. This testing is definitive for establishing the diagnosis and is widely commercially available. Liver biopsy used to be the gold-standard for diagnosis, but is now more often used to confirm the diagnosis when only one *HFE* mutation can be identified in a patient with evidence of iron overload or to detect whether cirrhosis is present.

Progress towards therapy

There is no consensus whether population-based biochemical and/or genetic screening programmes should be implemented to identify presymptomatic patients. However, patients at high risk due to family history (e.g. all first-degree relatives of a patient with confirmed hereditary haemochromatosis), or those with evidence of excess iron should be tested. Regular phlebotomy provides an effective treatment of iron overload to prevent end-organ damage, but does not reverse existing pathology.

Mucopolysaccharidosis (MPS) type I (Hurler, Scheie or Hurler/Scheie syndromes)

Clinical features

Symptoms of this lysosomal storage disorder are secondary to deposition of incompletely degraded mucopolysaccharides (glycosaminoglycans) in cellular lysosomes of numerous tissues including the brain, liver and cardiac valves. There is a broad range in disease severity, and at the most severe end of the spectrum patients are diagnosed with Hurler syndrome. Clinical disease starts during the first two years of life and is progressive with coarse facial features, clouding of the cornea, short stature, skeletal abnormalities (dysostosis multiplex), hepatosplenomegaly and mental retardation. Death occurs by age 10 years in untreated patients. At the attenuated end of the spectrum is Scheie syndrome, a slowly progressive disease without mental retardation and with a relatively normal lifespan.

Gene and disease-related gene product

The *IDUA* gene (4p16.3) codes for the enzyme α-L-iduronidase, deficiency of which leads to accumulation of incompletely degraded mucopolysaccarides. Seventy-five mutations in *IDUA* have been identified and for certain mutations genotype–phenotype prognostication is possible.

Diagnosis

The presence of an MPS disorder can be identified on a urinary screening test (such as a Berry spot) that identifies elevated gylcosaminoglycans in the urine. Definitive testing requires demonstration of decreased cellular α-L-iduronidase enzyme activity and/or detection of common mutations by targeted mutation analysis. Gene sequencing can also be performed to look for uncommon mutations.

Progress towards therapy

Bone marrow transplantation (BMT) has proven to be an effective therapy, though the broad range in disease severity complicates interpretation of its efficacy. Cognitive impairment cannot be reversed by BMT, so transplantation is most effective if performed early. Weekly enzyme replacement, with recombinant human α-L-iduronidase, reverses hepatosplenomegaly and improves generalized well-being so it is likely to become a standard adjunct to BMT. As the enzyme does not cross the blood–brain barrier, new treatments, such as neural stem cells, that can prevent and/or reverse brain pathology are under investigation.

Phenylketonuria

Clinical features

Phenylketonuria (PKU) is an inborn error of metabolism resulting from the failure to metabolize phenylalanine to tyrosine. Increased blood levels of L-phenylalanine lead to mental retardation, while hypopigmentation of the skin and hair results from decreased tyrosine in untreated patients. Some preservation of enzyme function can be sufficient to prevent mental retardation. High levels of phenylalanine in pregnant women with PKU are teratogenic (*see* Box "Teratogen", p 110) and can cause microcephaly and congenital heart disease in the developing foetus.

Gene and disease-related gene product

Phenylalanine hydroxylase, encoded for by *PAH* (12q22–24) converts the amino acid phenylalanine to tyrosine, which is required for dopamine synthesis. Over 400 different mutations have been identified, so most patients are compound heterozygotes, that is, possess two different disease alleles. Numerous mutations have arisen independently throughout Europe so that there is no single common European mutation.

Diagnosis

Initially, the diagnosis was made by the 'mousy' smell of urine in affected patients (due to the presence of phenylketones, a by-product of phenylalanine metabolism). Phenylketonuria was the first condition for which mass newborn screening was implemented. An increased phenylalanine level can be detected by one of several screening assays. The Guthrie bacterial inhibition test, performed on a blood spot obtained from neonates, was used initially for screening but has been replaced in many centres by tandem mass spectrometry. Definitive diagnosis is based on quantitative amino acid analysis and/or mutation detection, though the latter is not done routinely in clinical practice.

Progress towards therapy

With lifelong adherence to a reduced phenylalanine diet, essentially normal development ensues, though affected patients may have lower IQs than their non-affected siblings. Relaxation of dietary restriction after childhood has been associated with mild cognitive decline and behavioural problems. Women who may become pregnant should remain on a phenylalanine restricted diet to reduce the risk of foetal damage. The severely restrictive diet can be relaxed in some individuals by pharmacologic doses of biopterin, a vitamin cofactor of the phenylalanine hydroxylase enzyme. Gene therapy using both viral and non-viral vectors has been tried but results in PKU animal models are not yet encouraging.

> **Teratogen**
>
> A teratogen is an agent (drug, substance, exposure) that interferes with normal embryonic development, resulting in abnormalities of structure or function. Less thaen 5% of congenital malformations are known to be caused by a teratogen.

Spinal muscular atrophy

Clinical features

Spinal muscular atrophy (SMA) is a neurodegenerative disorder with progressive weakness due to motor neuron loss of the anterior horn cells in the spinal cord and brainstem. It is relatively common, affecting ~1/10 000 liveborns and the carrier frequency is as high as 1/50. By some estimates, SMA is the leading genetic cause of infant mortality. It is clinically divided into three subtypes: type I presents with severe hypotonia and weakness during infancy and a respiratory death usually ensues by two years of age; type II has onset of symptoms before two years of age, and although children acquire some motor milestones, most never walk independently; and type III has the mildest course with later onset and survival into adulthood.

Gene and disease-related gene product

All types of SMA are caused by deletions involving both copies of the survival motor neuron 1 (*SMN1*) gene (*5q13*). The ubiquitously expressed gene product, SMN1, forms part of a complex important for the assembly of small nuclear ribonucleoproteins. Deletions in *SMN1* interfere with normal mRNA processing and by an as yet unknown mechanism harm motor neuron survival. Normal survival of motor neurons requires the presence of at least one functioning copy of *SMN1*.

The variable phenotype of SMA is explained, in part, by the presence of an *SMN2* gene, adjacent to the *SMN1* gene. These two genes have very high sequence homology, with only five base pair differences. In the most serious type of SMA, one or both copies of *SMN2* are missing, whereas milder and later-onset SMA is associated with three or four copies of the *SMN2* gene arising from gene duplication. Thus, the *SMN2* protein product compensates for *SMN1* efficiency and influences the SMA phenotype.

Diagnosis

The diagnosis is suggested by weakness, absent deep tendon reflexes and characteristically abnormal electromyography (EMG, which records the electrical activity of muscle). The diagnosis is confirmed in 95% of patients by demonstrating loss of exons 7 and 8 in both copies of the *SMN1* gene. The most widely used testing method, available in commercial laboratories, is PCR–RFLP which is able to distinguish *SMN1* from *SMN2*. Sibling recurrence risk is usually 25% as both parents are likely to be carriers. However, *de novo* deletions in the *SMN1* gene can occur, so that the carrier status of both parents should be confirmed using quantitative PCR-RFLP.

Progress towards therapy

Therapy at the present time is supportive with particular attention to optimizing respiratory status. Techniques to up-regulate and stabilize the full length *SMN2* gene product, in an attempt to compensate for abnormal or absent *SMN1* gene product, continue to be investigated. Greater understanding of the particular sensitivity shown by motor neurons to decreased SMN protein levels may also provide clues for future therapies.

Wilson disease (Hepatolenticular degeneration)

Clinical features

A disorder of copper metabolism, affecting ~1/30 000 individuals, Wilson disease is characterized by toxic copper deposition in the liver, brain and cornea. In ~40% of cases, symptoms develop between childhood and young adulthood, generally starting with liver disease (hepatitis, jaundice or hepatic failure). The remainder of cases present between adolescence and adulthood, principally with neuropsychiatric symptoms (e.g. movement disorders, dystonia, depression or cognitive deterioration). A common finding independent of the mode of presentation is a Kayser–Fleischer ring which is a visible copper deposit in the cornea of the eye.

Gene and disease-related gene product

Copper is a cofactor for a number of important enzymes. The body must rid itself of excess copper and the protein copper-transporting ATPase2, coded for by the *ATP7B* gene (13q14.2-21), plays important roles in this process. ATPase2 helps copper bind to the major copper transporter, ceruloplasmin, and is also involved in biliary excretion of excess copper. Abnormal accumulation of cellular copper leads to oxidative damage and cell death.

Diagnosis

Diagnosis is suggested by low serum copper and ceruloplasmin levels, presence of Kayser–Fleischer rings, elevated urinary copper, and ultrastructural changes on liver biopsy. Genetic analysis of *ATP7B* is commercially available for common mutations, which account for 60% of the abnormal alleles in British populations. Over 200 mutations have been identified, so that most affected individuals are compound heterozygotes (i.e. have a different mutation in each copy of *ATP7B*). Exon or gene sequencing can be performed to identify rare mutations. If both mutations cannot be identified in a person with Wilson disease, linkage analysis can be used to identify at-risk family members and/or gene carriers.

Progress towards therapy

Standard therapy involves copper chelation with agents such as penicillamine and maintenance treatment with high doses of zinc. Liver transplantation is offered when advanced liver failure is present. The introduction of the human *ATP7B* gene into a rodent model of Wilson disease resulted in significant improvement in copper homeostasis and reversal of hepatic dysfunction.

X-linked disorders

Duchenne muscular dystrophy

Clinical features

Duchenne muscular dystrophy (DMD) is the most common X-linked neuromuscular disorder, affecting ~1/3500 liveborn males. Phenotypically, males are normal at birth but show delayed motor milestones and manifest obvious skeletal muscle weakness by two to five years of age. Creatine phosphokinase (CK) levels are 5–10 times the upper limit of normal, even in presymptomatic young infants. Abnormal findings that develop include pseudohypertrophy of the calf muscles and proximal weakness. Progressive weakness ensues and most males are wheelchair bound by their teenage years and deceased by their mid-twenties. Dilated cardiomyopathy eventually develops in all affected males. Less than 20% of female carriers demonstrate muscle weakness, though up to half have mild to moderate serum CK elevations. A milder disorder, Becker muscular dystrophy, is now known to be allelic to Duchenne muscular dystrophy (*see* below).

Gene and disease-related gene product

The *DMD* gene (Xp21.2) codes for the cytoskeletal protein dystrophin. *DMD* is one of the largest genes in the human genome encompassing 79 exons. Its large size may predispose to the occurrence of many genetic alterations, most often deletions and duplications, but point and splice site mutations also occur. It is, therefore, not surprising that a mutation in *DMD* arises *de novo* in ~1/3 of all affected males. The *DMD* gene codes for the protein dystrophin, a component of a multi-protein dystrophin-associated complex. The role of this complex is to link the intracellular actin cytoskeleton to the extracellular matrix, providing sarcolemma stability during muscle contractions. The mechanism by which abnormal or absent dystrophin leads to membrane damage and ultimately, muscle destruction is not entirely clear. In males with DMD, the genetic changes in the *DMD* gene are 'out-of-frame', resulting in dystrophin protein that is either absent or severely truncated. In Becker muscular dystrophy, however, the *DMD* gene changes are 'in-frame', resulting in partially functional dystrophin protein that is either reduced in amount or size.

Diagnosis

Elevated CK suggests the diagnosis of a muscular dystrophy. Histologic examination of a muscle biopsy specimen reveals non-specific and non-diagnostic muscle changes. However, dystrophin staining by immunohistochemistry is diagnostic, as the staining is either absent or in a patchy distribution. Most often, the diagnosis is established by molecular genetic testing. Approximately two-third of patients have a deletion in the *DMD* gene, which can be detected by PCR, Southern blot analysis, and/or FISH. These methods for deletion detection are widely available. Mutation testing in female carriers and sequencing for uncommon or point mutations tends to be restricted to specialty DNA diagnostic laboratories.

Progress towards therapy

In addition to supportive treatment such as physical therapy, prednisone improves muscle strength and function by a currently unknown mechanism. However, the side effects of daily steroids are considerable. Numerous attempts to introduce a functioning copy of the *DMD* gene have been made and new studies are underway. However, effective gene therapy is difficult due to the large number of affected muscle cells that need to be targeted, and the large size of *DMD* (over 2 Mbp), which is beyond the capacity of retroviral vectors. Non-viral vectors, such as plasmids, can deliver the large-sized gene, but are not efficient at gaining entry into muscle cells. A technique that involves delivering truncated forms of the *DMD* gene (dystrophin minigenes) encoding smaller, yet functional, proteins is effective in treating an animal model of Duchenne muscular dystrophy, the *mdx* mouse. Unfortunately, human DMD is far more severe than disease in the *mdx* mouse, so the utility of this technique in humans remains unknown. One final promising technique worthy of mention is that of antisense induced exon skipping. Its premise is to enlarge an 'out-of-frame' deletion to an 'in-frame' deletion (i.e. converting a

Duchenne phenotype to a Becker phenotype). This has been accomplished by use of antisense oligonucleotides in cultured muscle cells from both the *mdx* mouse and from male patients with Duchenne muscular dystrophy.

Fabry disease

Clinical features

Fabry disease is a lysosomal disorder in which certain sphingolipid moieties accumulate in the endothelial cell lining of blood vessels, smooth muscle cells, myocardium of the heart and glomeruli of the kidneys. Early onset strokes are the most serious clinical manifestation of Fabry disease and these occur in up to 25% of affected males. The cause of strokes appears to be either due to endothelial cells swollen with non-degradable sphingolipids occluding the vessel lumen, or damage to the vessel wall resulting in aneurysmal thinning and dilatation. The average age of stroke onset is 36 years in males. Presenting symptoms that often start in childhood include acute or chronic 'burning' pain of the hands and feet lasting minutes to days or even weeks, characteristic skin lesions known as angiokeratomas (clusters of non-blanching dilated small blood vessels which are dark red in colour) and corneal opacities detected on slit-lamp examination. Later features due to continued sphingolipid accumulation are cardiac problems (such as cardiomyopathy, myocardial infarction and arrhythmias) and renal disease due to deposition of sphingolipid in the glomeruli. Mental retardation and facial dysmorphology do not occur in Fabry disease. Life expectancy is reduced in untreated patients, secondary to recurrent strokes and cardiac or renal failure. There is a broad spectrum of disease severity in carrier females, ranging from clinically normal to severe disease, including stroke and renal failure. An increasing number of cardiac and renal Fabry disease variants are being recognized, in which patients have higher residual enzyme activity and primarily manifest cardiac or renal involvement.

Gene and disease-related gene product

Over 300 mutations in the *GLA* gene (Xq22), which codes for alpha-galactosidase A, have been identified to date. Most mutations are unique to each family.

Diagnosis

The diagnosis of Fabry disease is established in specialized biochemistry laboratories by demonstrating decreased enzyme activity of alpha-galactosidase A in plasma, white blood cells or fibroblasts. In males, Fabry disease is usually associated with <1% alpha-galactosidase A activity, while patients with the cardiac variant have 10% activity. Enzyme activity cannot be reliably used to identify female carriers. Sequencing of the *GLA* gene identifies mutations in almost all affected males and most carrier females; this testing is clinically available in selected DNA diagnostic laboratories.

Progress towards therapy

Antiplatelet drugs are administered in an attempt to prevent stroke, anti-coagulants are used to treat strokes that are thrombo-embolic, and analgesics are needed to control the extremity pain. Dialysis or kidney transplantation is done to treat renal failure. Infusion of human recombinant alpha-galactoside A enzyme is very effective and leads to improved cerebral blood flow, stabilization of renal disease, and reversal of cardiac pathology. Even though the cost of treatment is ~160 000 euros/year, enzyme replacement treatment is now the therapy of choice and should be offered to all males with a confirmed diagnosis of Fabry disease, preferably before symptoms develop. Current recommendations are that enzyme replacement therapy should be given only to symptomatic females. Gene therapy using a viral vector to introduce a normally functioning copy of alpha-galactosidase A in a mouse model of Fabry disease successfully lowered the level of accumulated sphingolipid; in the future, gene therapy may replace enzyme replacement therapy as the treatment of choice.

Haemophilia

Clinical features

A common clotting disorder, haemophilia affects 1/4000 liveborn males, and is due most often to deficiency of either factor VIII (haemophilia A or classical haemophilia) or factor IX (haemophilia B or Christmas disease). Half of affected males have a positive family history. The most famous haemophilia family is that of Queen Victoria, whose carrier daughters married into the Russian and Spanish royal houses. Excess bleeding occurs due to insufficient thrombin formation to stabilize the fibrin clot. Disease severity corresponds to the level of factor activity. For classic haemophilia, <1% activity is found in severely affected patients, who suffer spontaneous bleeding into joints and soft tissues and excessive bleeding in response to trauma or surgery. 5–35% activity is typically associated with prolonged bleeding following major trauma or surgery. Major sequelae in untreated patients include chronic joint disease from repeated bleeds and intracranial haemorrhage. Females carriers whose factor activity level is <35% are at risk for bleeding following major surgery.

Genes and disease-related gene products

Males with haemophilia A, which comprises ~80% of cases, have a mutation in the factor VIII gene (*F8*, Xq28), while those with haemophilia B have a mutation in the factor IX (*F9*, Xq27) gene. The factor VIII gene contains 26 exons and within exon 22 are two nested genes (factor VIII A & B) that are of unknown function; additional copies of the A gene are located nearby. These multiple copies of the factor VIII A gene increase the likelihood of homologous recombination; the single most common mutation producing severe haemophilia A involves an inversion in intron 22 with subsequent separation of exons 1–22 from exons 23–26. Other genetic changes

such as deletions, insertions and a variety of point mutations underlie the remaining cases.

Diagnosis

Routinely available coagulation tests are usually normal in patients with haemophilia A, though partial thromboplastin time (PTT) may be prolonged in severe cases. Specific assays of factors VIII and IX must be performed to establish the diagnosis. Additionally, other bleeding disorders, such as von Willebrand disease (*see* p 100), must be ruled out. Mutation analysis, to detect the common intron 22 inversion, or gene sequencing to detect other mutations, is widely available. Genetic testing can confirm the diagnosis in affected males and can also detect carrier females and affected foetuses as part of prenatal diagnosis. Linkage analysis can also determine disease status in familial cases where a mutation has not been identified by sequencing.

Progress towards therapy

Standard treatment for haemophilia A involves infusion of factor VIII concentrate. Prior to the availability of recombinant factors, factors were obtained from pooled human plasma so that a high proportion of haemophiliacs contracted hepatitis or HIV, increasing the death rate from treatment-related complications over that due to disease-related complications. Milder cases of haemophilia A can be treated with DDAVP (desmopressin, a synthetic antidiuretic hormone) as this raises factor VIII levels. The lack of requirement for tissue-specific expression or precise regulation of the deficient factors (small amounts have significant clinical benefits and large amounts do not appear harmful) make haemophilia an excellent candidate for gene therapy. Examples of human therapy trials include: implantation of autologous skin fibroblasts transfected with a modified factor VIII which led to mild increases in factor VIII levels for about one year; retrovirus or 'gutless' adenovirus vectors, though the latter vector has been complicated by immune reactions and transient elevations of liver transaminases;

and a new class of vectors, recombinant adeno-associated viral vectors (rAAV), which shows considerable promise for transduction of the factor IX gene, but the large size of the factor VIII gene will require modifications in the method of gene delivery.

Mucopolysaccharidosis type II (Hunter syndrome, MPS II)

Clinical features

A lysosomal storage disease, similar to the autosomal recessive MPS I (Hurler syndrome) though generally less severe. The phenotype of Hunter syndrome is similar to that of Hurler syndrome, though the corneas remain clear. Life expectancy is shortened, and survival beyond 15 years of age is unlikely.

Gene and disease-related gene product

Numerous mutations in the gene, *IDS* (Xq28.2), result in a deficiency of the enzyme iduronate 2-sulphatase.

Diagnosis

The same diagnostic strategy discussed for MPS I (Hurler syndrome) (*see* p 109) is applicable. The diagnosis is confirmed by finding either mutations in *IDS* and/or decreased activity of iduronate 2-sulphatase in cultured fibroblasts.

Progress towards therapy

Bone marrow transplantation ameliorates the physical manifestation of Hunter syndrome but has no effect on reversing or stabilizing the mental retardation. Enzyme activity has been restored in lymphoblastoid cells and CD34+ stem cells from patients with Hunter syndrome that have been transduced with a retroviral vector containing the iduronate 2-sulphatase gene. Gene therapy trials are underway.

Wiskott–Aldrich syndrome and X-linked thrombocytopenia

Clinical features

In affected males, classic Wiskott–Aldrich syndrome is characterized by eczema, thrombocytopenia and defects of the immune system. Thrombocytopenia is present at birth and can be life-threatening; the platelets are small in size. Recurrent pneumonias and sinus infections are very common. Most affected males have eczema, though the extent of skin lesions is highly variable. Additional problems involving autoimmune disease and malignancy (such as Epstein–Barr virus B cell lymphoma) can develop over time. Female heterozygote carriers preferentially inactivate the X chromosome bearing the Wiskott–Aldrich mutation in their blood cells, so they show no manifestations of the disorder. X-linked thrombocytopenia, characterized by thrombocytopenia and small platelet size, is now known to be allelic to Wiskott–Aldrich syndrome.

Gene and disease-related gene product

The *WAS* gene (Xp11) codes for the Wiskott–Aldrich syndrome protein (WASp). Several hundred different mutations have been identified to date, and relatively good genotype–phenotype correlations exist. Specifically, missense mutations are associated with mild disease, while mutations that eliminate a functional protein product are associated with severe disease. WASp plays an important role in the cytoskeleton of the cell, directly binding to actin and supporting actin filament branching.

Diagnosis

Males are diagnosed based on the constellation of medical problems and laboratory findings; thrombocytopenia is the most consistent abnormality. Clinically available sequencing of the *WAS* gene detects almost all mutations in affected males and carrier females. Targeted mutation screening for selected exons is widely available.

Progress towards therapy

At present bone marrow transplantation is the treatment of choice for severe cases and best results come from HLA-matched sibling donors. Transfused blood products, that contain white blood cells, must be irradiated to prevent graft versus host disease. Splenectomy may increase platelet count but is also likely to increase the risk of infections. Using a Wiskott–Aldrich mouse model, retroviral transduction has successfully restored expression of normal WASp in haemopoietic stem cells. Gene therapy may be a possible treatment option for affected persons with this disorder in the future.

X-linked adrenoleucodystrophy (Cerebral adrenoleucodystrophy and adrenomyeloneuropathy)

Clinical features

This is the disorder that afflicted Lorenzo Odone, whose story was told in the film *Lorenzo's Oil*. X-linked adrenoleucodystrophy is one of a family of disorders of the peroxisome, a cellular organelle that metabolizes very long chain fatty acids, among other tasks. Affected males accumulate saturated very long chain fatty acids in their brain and adrenal glands. Resulting symptoms include cerebral demyelination, progressive neurological disability and adrenal insufficiency. In young males, the disorder presents with progressive neurological symptoms such as spasticity, seizures, visual loss and dementia (so-called cerebral adrenoleucodystrophy). Presentation in teenage or adult males (referred to adrenomyeloneuropathy) is primarily that of a spinal disorder including gait, sphincter, and erectile disturbances, though cognitive or behavioural deterioration can occur as well. Disease severity can differ significantly even among members of the same family. MRI scans of the brain demonstrate demyelination, especially in childhood presentations of the disorder. Female carriers can develop spasticity of the lower extremities and urinary incontinence in middle age; in the absence of a positive family history, females can mistakenly be diagnosed as having multiple sclerosis.

Gene and disease-related gene product

The gene responsible for this disorder is *ABCD1* (Xq28). *ABCD1* encodes a member of the ATP-binding cassette protein transporter family, a group of proteins important for transporting molecules across cell membranes. The central nervous system and adrenal cortex are the sites where very long chain fatty acid metabolism normally takes place. In affected males, long chain fatty acids accumulate in these organs, alter membrane stability and through undefined mechanisms lead to cellular damage. Additionally, an inflammatory response that destroys myelin occurs in the childhood presentation of the disorder. Over 500 mutations have been identified in the *ABCD1* gene, and a private, or unique, mutation is found in most families.

Diagnosis

A specialized biochemistry laboratory can reliably establish the diagnosis in affected males by plasma determination of very long chain fatty acids, which show characteristic patterns of elevation. However, biochemical testing is reliable in diagnosing only 85% of female carriers. Mutation detection in *ABCD1*, by either direct sequencing or Southern blot analysis, can be used to confirm the diagnosis, but most often is used for detecting female carriers and for prenatal diagnosis of foetuses at risk for inheriting the disorder.

Progress towards therapy

If adrenal insufficiency is present, steroid supplementation is required but this treatment has no impact on neurological symptoms. Lorenzo's oil, a 4 : 1 mixture of glyceryl-trioleate and glyceryl trierucate, is able to normalize very long chain fatty acid levels in plasma, but its clinical efficacy remains unclear. Bone marrow transplantation is effective, but should be reserved for males early in the course of the cerebral form of the disorder. Overexpression of a highly homologous gene, *ABCD2*, ameliorated the phenotype in a transgenic mouse with abnormalities similar to human adrenomyeloneuropathy and may be a model for human gene therapy.

X-linked Alport syndrome

Clinical features

Alport syndrome encompasses disorders with progressive renal disease, hearing impairment and ocular abnormalities. These abnormalities are caused by defects in collagen proteins, a constituent of basement membranes on which epithelial cells attach. Alport syndrome is estimated to affect 1/50 000 persons and accounts for 3% of paediatric renal failure, but <1% of adult renal failure. Approximately 80% of all cases are due to the X-linked form of the disorder. Affected males are more severely affected than carrier females. Males present during childhood with microscopic haematuria (red blood cells in urine seen on microscopic examination), episodes of gross or visible haematuria and mild hearing loss detectable on formal audiologic evaluation. Proteinuria and hypertension develop over time. By 30–40 years of age, all males have clinically significant renal dysfunction or end-stage-renal-disease and sensorineural hearing loss; ~1/3 have ocular abnormalities, such as anterior lenticonus (anterior displacement of the lens of the eye), and pigmentary retinopathy, findings which are almost pathognomonic for Alport syndrome. Many female carriers have intermittent haematuria though only a small minority progress to significant renal disease; almost half develop sensorineural hearing loss.

Gene and disease-related gene product

Alport syndrome is due to mutations in collagen genes. Normal collagen proteins interact with other proteins to form the structural components of basement membranes. X-linked Alport syndrome is due to mutations in the *COL4A5* gene (Xq22.3). Mutations lead to translation of either deficient or abnormal type IV collagen alpha chain 5. Basement membrane pathology develops over time and is responsible for the disease manifestations described above. Several hundred mutations in the *COL4A5* gene have been identified to date. Examples of mutations include those that delete a portion of the gene or point mutations leading to replacement of a glycine (every third amino acid) by a bulkier or charged amino acid (*see* Osteogenesis Imperfecta, p 97, for further details). Deletions within the *COL4A5* gene and nonsense mutations consistently lead to earlier onset end-stage-renal-disease, while missense mutations do not prognohsticate onset of renal failure.

Diagnosis

The diagnosis of Alport syndrome can be established by a renal biopsy, revealing a characteristic appearance of abnormal glomerular basement membranes by electron microscopy. Antibody staining for the alpha 5 chain of type 4 collagen will be absent in the glomerular and tubular basement membranes of affected males, while carrier females will demonstrate patchy staining. The diagnosis can be established by less invasive methods. Specifically, absence of staining for the alpha 5 chain of type 4 collagen in a skin sample confirms the diagnosis of X-linked Alport syndrome in males. Finally, genetic analysis of the *COL4A5* gene is also available to establish the diagnosis, though this is not straightforward given the many different mutations identified to date. Gene sequencing can be performed on a clinical basis, in selected DNA diagnostic laboratories.

Progress towards therapy

Kidney transplantation is the most successful method of treating renal failure in Alport syndrome. However, in some cases, transplant recipients make antibodies against the normal collagen protein in the donor kidney since they are not tolerant to this protein; this results in anti-glomerular basement membrane nephritis. Gene therapy will require delivering a normal collagen gene to the proper location in the kidney. In a canine model of Alport syndrome, a normal collagen gene transduced (*see* p 44, 80) using an adenoviral vector was successfully expressed within the glomeruli following direct renal perfusion. Additional studies are needed to determine the longevity of normal gene expression.

Conditions attributed to mutations in two or more different genes

A few of the disorders described above are caused by mutations in different genes. For example, 80% of cases with Alport syndrome (*see* p 117) are X-linked caused by mutations in *COL4A5*. The remainder of cases are autosomal recessive or autosomal dominant due to mutations in other collagen genes. Similarly, 90% of cases with Congenital Adrenal Hyperplasia (*see* p 103) are caused by mutations in the gene coding for the 21-hydroxylase enzyme; the remaining cases are due to other mutations interfering with the normal synthesis of cortisol. However, there are important genetic conditions where no single gene accounts for the majority of cases; rather there is extensive genetic heterogeneity (i.e. mutations in numerous different genes producing a similar phenotype). Examples of several of these conditions are presented below.

Hirschsprung disease

Hirschsprung disease is a neural crest disorder leading to functional gastrointestinal obstruction affecting 1/5000 births. The underlying defect involves absence of ganglion cells in the distal hindgut so that affected infants present with intestinal blockage. Most cases have short-segment Hirschsprung disease due to absence, or diminished number, of ganglion cells in the sigmoid colon while the minority have long-segment disease due to more widespread reduction in the number of ganglion cells. Males are four times more likely to be affected than females. Although Hirschsprung disease occurs as an isolated problem is most cases, it can occur in association with chromosome abnormalities, such as Down syndrome, or as part of several single gene disorders. Following improved diagnostic recognition as well as surgical techniques to treat the disorder, it was apparent that Hirschsprung clustered in families in an autosomal dominant pattern of inheritance with incomplete penetrance (*see* Box "Penetrance", p 108) and variable expressivity.

Using both linkage analysis techniques and candidate gene cloning, mutations in the *RET* proto-oncogene have been identified as the cause of Hirschsprung in ~30–40% of cases. *RET* is a transmembrane receptor with an intracellular tyrosine kinase domain; it is expressed in neural crest cells and normally plays a role in promoting cell growth and differentiation. Interestingly, mutations in *RET* associated with Hirschsprung disease are *loss* of function mutations. *Gain* of function mutations in *RET* cause a distinct phenotype, Multiple Endocrine Neoplasia 2 (MEN2); this entity is most often associated with medullary thyroid carcinoma, pheochromocytoma and parathyroid hyperplasia or adenoma.

Mutations in *RET* account for <50% of cases with Hirschsprung disease. When a mutation in *RET* is identified, first-degree relatives should be offered mutation analysis as well, even if they are asymptomatic because incomplete penetrance is well-documented. This testing is widely available. Mutations have also been identified in several other genes such as the ligand and co-receptor for *RET* as well as in a completely non-related pathway, the endothelin receptor and its ligand; clinical testing is not available for these genes.

Hypertrophic cardiomyopathy

Hypertrophic cardiomyopathy (HCM) is defined on echocardiography as (asymmetric) thickening of the wall of the left ventricle along with a decrease in the size of the left ventricular cavity, which are not caused primarily by hypertension or left ventricular outflow obstruction. Presenting symptoms are very diverse including: syncope (fainting), anginal chest pain, arrhythmias and sudden death especially in young athletes. However, some patients never demonstrate any symptoms. Patients who have compromised left-ventricular outflow with diminished aortic output have greater risk for disease progression and sudden death. HCM is a very common cardiac disorder affecting ~1/500 persons and follows an autosomal dominant pattern of inheritance. It is caused by mutations in a dozen different genes that code for proteins involved in the structure or function of the cardiac sarcomere (cardiac muscle cell unit bounded by Z bands, seen on light microscopy). The most common mutations are those that affect the sarcomere thick or thin filaments, involving the cardiac beta-myosin heavy chain, myosin-binding protein C and cardiac troponin-T. Most mutations are missense mutations and are unique to each family. Given the presence of considerable clinical variability between affected members of the same family, additional genetic or non-genetic factors must also affect the phenotype. Since HCM almost always is an autosomal dominant disorder, first degree relatives of an affected individual should be screened for the presence of HCM, by an echocardiogram or genetic testing. Testing for some of the more common mutations is commercially available, whereas testing for some of the less common mutations is offered in specialized research laboratories. Beta-blockers effectively treat symptoms such as chest pain; anti-arrhythmics are indicated in some patients. A small percent of patients require surgery involving removal of hypertrophied heart muscle (myomectomy). The most effective therapy for decreasing the risk from sudden death is implantation of a cardioverter-defibrillator. Recombinant adeno-associated virus (rAAV) has successfully transduced myocytes in animal models and may offer hope for gene therapy in the future.

Retinitis pigmentosa

The Retinitis pigmentosas (RPs) are a group of disorders that produce retinal degeneration and visual loss. Collectively, RPs are common, affecting ~1/5000 persons, but numerous individual subtypes exist. Initial symptoms are night blindness due to loss of rods photoreceptors, constriction of visual fields, retinal pigment changes and attenuation of retinal blood vessels. Eventual death of cone photoreceptors occurs so that daytime vision and central visual field loss develop over time. RP can occur as part of multi-system syndromes, but most often it is the only abnormality in the affected individual. Half of cases follow clear-cut autosomal dominant, autosomal recessive, or X-linked patterns of inheritance. The remainder are classified as 'sporadic' and probably represent new dominant mutations or the first affected member of an autosomal recessive kindred. Age of onset varies considerably from infancy to adulthood. Over 35 different genes have been identified which result in RP and no single gene accounts for the majority of cases. Gene function falls into several categories such as photoreceptor structure, retinal development and RNA splicing. The most common gene responsible for autosomal dominant RP, the Rhodopsin (*RHO*) gene, plays a major role in the visual cascade of converting light into a neuronal signal; over 100 different mutations in *RHO* have been identified to date. A discussion of the many genes responsible for RP is beyond the scope of this text. RP is diagnosed by direct ophthalmologic examination, electroretinography, visual field testing and family history. Molecular testing for a dozen of the known RP genes is clinically available; testing for additional genes is available in selected research laboratories. There is no cure for RP. Daily supplementation with 15 000 IU vitamin A may slow disease progression, but excess vitamin A must be avoided as toxicities can occur. Gene therapy has shown promise in animal models with retinal degeneration; growth factors that slow death of photoreceptors have been successfully transduced into photoreceptor cells and retinal pigment epithelium, following direct retinal or subretinal injection of the viral vector.

Trinucleotide (TNT) repeat disorders

The genetic basis for several disorders with prominent neurologic or neurodegenerative features is an increased number of trinucleotide repeats, most commonly $(CAG)_n$. Trinucleotide (TNT) repeat disorders are generally inherited in an autosomal dominant or X-linked pattern.

Effect of CAG Repeats

CAG codes for the amino acid glutamine. A string of CAGs → a series of glutamines, a so-called Polyglutamine tract.

Due to the possibility of expansion in the number of repeats during meiosis, TNT disorders demonstrate 'anticipation' with earlier symptom onset in successive generations (*see* Chapter 2, p 55). There are two types of TNT disorders depending on whether or not the repeats are translated into the protein product. In the first type, the expanded repeat segment lies within the coding region of the gene and the additional amino acids become incorporated into the protein as a long series of glutamines, forming a polyglutamine tract. The resulting protein may engage in abnormal folding and/or abnormal protein–protein interactions, forming intracellular aggregates that ultimately are toxic to the cell. In the second type, the triplet repeat is in a non-coding region of the gene, and hence is not translated. The mechanisms by which these untranslated TNT repeats lead to disease are not entirely clear but symptoms may be due to disordered DNA structure and/or aberrant RNA synthesis.

For each of these disorders, the repeat size falls into one of three categories: (1) normal range: repeat size is stable during cell division; individuals carrying this repeat size are normal; (2) intermediate or premutation range: repeat size may expand during meiosis, so there is increased risk for having an offspring with a full mutation; individuals carrying this repeat size may either be normal or have mild abnormalities, depending on the specific disorder; or (3) full mutation range: repeat size has expanded beyond a normal or premutation threshold so that individuals are affected with the disorder (*see* Box "Premuation versus Full mutation"). The size of the repeat that leads to disease varies among the different disorders.

Diagnosis

TNT repeat disorders are diagnosed by genetic testing to quantify the repeat size by PCR or by Southern blotting, in the case of large repeats.

Treatment

Treatment of all known TNT repeat disorders is symptomatic with medical management of existing symptoms and problems. Clinical trials are underway to identify medications to slow the progression of medical and neurological problems.

Premutation Versus Full Mutation

Both categories indicate the presence of greater than the normal number of trinucleotide repeats. Premutation carriers are phenotypically normal themselves, or manifest mild and/or late onset disease-related problems. However, their triplet repeat size can expand during meiosis resulting in a full mutation and a phenotypically abnormal individual.

Fragile X syndrome

Clinical features

Fragile X syndrome, also referred to as FRAXA, is the most common inherited mental retardation syndrome. Approximately 1/5000 males and ~1/8000 females have a full mutation (>200 CGG repeats) in the gene responsible for Fragile X syndrome. In affected males, mental retardation and behavioural problems, such as impulsivity and short attention span, are universal. Autistic-like features are common as well. Among females who carry a full mutation, half have mental retardation or significant learning disabilities. The presence of the second normal X chromosome in females presumably ameliorates the phenotype. Cognitive deterioration is not a feature of Fragile X syndrome. There are no or only subtle physical manifestations in the pre-pubertal period, but post-pubertal males tend to have a long, narrow face, prominent ears, and macro-orchidism (enlarged testicles). A mild connective tissue dysplasia, leading to joint laxity and mitral valve prolapse is also common.

The number of individuals who have a premutation is much greater than the number who have a full mutation; *premutations* are estimated to be present in 1/200–1/500 females and ~1/1500 males. Initial observations were that most premutation carriers were phenotypically normal, but there is growing evidence to refute this. Among premutation carrier females, 20% have premature ovarian failure and an even greater number have subclinical ovarian failure. Additionally, there is an increased risk for emotional difficulties such as anxiety and perseveration. Among males, recent observations demonstrate that as many as one-third of elderly premutation males will develop progressive tremor and ataxia, so-called Fragile-X-associated tremor/ataxia syndrome.

Gene and disease-related gene product

The genetic defect is an expansion of a triplet repeat (CGG) in the 5′ untranslated region of the gene *FMR1,* located near the end of the long arm of the X chromosome (Xq27.3). *FMR1* codes for a protein named FMRP, fragile X mental retardation protein, which is highly expressed in the brain. Its normal function is to bind specific classes of RNA and regulate protein synthesis in neurons. A full mutation is associated methylation of *FMR1* and subsequent gene silencing, so that no FMRP product is translated. The absence of FMRP determines the phenotype interfering with normal synapse and dendrite formation. Expansion from a premutation to a full mutation only takes place during oogenesis, and the larger the premutation, the greater the risk of expansion to a full mutation.

Diagnosis

Prior to the discovery of the *FMR1* gene, Fragile X syndrome in males was diagnosed by cytogenetic detection of a 'pinching in' (fragile site) at Xq27; the disorder was originally named for this observation. Diagnosis is now made by determination of the CGG repeat size in *FMR1.* Although there are some exceptions, normal repeat size is typically <59 CGG repeats, premutations range between 60 and 200 triplets, and Fragile X syndrome occurs when there are >200 CGG repeats. Repeat size is quantitated by PCR, though Southern blot analysis is needed for determining the size of larger repeats. This testing is widely available. Southern blotting can also determine the methylation status of the *FMR1* gene.

Progress towards therapy

Current therapy is supportive. An existing animal model of Fragile X syndrome, the *fmr1* mouse, does not accurately recapitulate the human phenotype. Genetic counselling is key for this disorder, as mothers of sons with Fragile X syndrome are either full mutation or premutation carriers themselves, and are at high risk for having more affected children. Additional family members are likely to be carriers as well.

Friedreich ataxia

Clinical features

Friedreich ataxia is an autosomal recessive disorder characterized by progressive ataxia (loss of coordination), loss of deep tendon reflexes, and hypertrophic cardiomyopathy. Symptoms typically develop before 25 years of age. It affects ~1/40 000 Caucasians and is much rarer in other ethnic groups. Neuropathology shows degeneration of sensory nerve dorsal root ganglia, spinocerebellar tracts and large peripheral sensory neurons. Disease onset occurs earlier in patients with a larger number of TNT repeats.

Gene and disease-related gene product

The *FRDA* gene (9q13) codes for the protein frataxin. This is a mitochondrial protein of poorly understood function, with an apparent role in the mitochondrial metabolism of iron and of oxygen. Triplet repeat expansion in the first intron of the gene leads to inhibition of transcription.

Diagnosis

A GAA intronic repeat in *FRDA* is expanded in 95% of affected persons. Since this is an autosomal recessive disorder, both copies of *FRDA* have abnormal GAA expansions in affected individuals. Commercially available testing, using either PCR or Southern blot, can determine the repeat size; direct sequencing can accurately determine the repeat length in premutation carriers.

Progress towards therapy

Frataxin has homology to a yeast protein (YFH1).* Study of this protein, which is involved in control of iron levels and cellular respiratory function, may help define the role of frataxin. Treatment is supportive but progression of the cardiomyopathy may be slowed by administration of a ubiquinone analogue (which functions as an antioxidant).

Huntington disease

Clinical features

Huntington disease is one of the best studied trinucleotide repeat disorders. It is an autosomal dominant condition characterized by progressive dementia, abnormal voluntary and involuntary movements and psychiatric disturbances. Chorea (involuntary brief irregular movements, especially of the extremities) develops in 90% of affected individuals. Survival is typically less than two decades following diagnosis. Although the mean age of onset is near 40 years of age, symptoms can develop before 20 or after 50 years. Larger repeat sizes are associated with earlier disease onset. Enlargement of the repeat size occurs only during spermatogenesis; accordingly, cases with juvenile onset Huntington disease will have inherited the mutation from their fathers. Most affected individuals have a positive family history; in other words, *de novo* cases of Huntington disease are rare.

Gene and disease-related gene product

The *HD* gene (4p16.3) normally contains up to 36 CAG trinucleotide repeats in exon 1; repeats of 27–35 fall into the intermediate or premutation range conferring no symptoms but an increased risk for expansion. Adult onset Huntington disease is generally found in individuals with repeat sizes between 36 and 55, while juvenile onset is typically found in persons with >60 repeats. *HD* codes for the protein, huntingtin. The protein is highly conserved across species, widely expressed in neurons throughout the brain, and appears to be unique without significant homology to other proteins. The exact mechanism by which the expanded polyglutamine tract in the huntingtin protein confers disease is not known, but the longer the repeat, the greater the number of abnormal neuronal intranuclear inclusions (though it is unclear if these inclusions are the cause, or the effect, of cell toxicity). Apoptosis is the mechanism underlying cell death and neurodegeneration.

Diagnosis

The diagnosis Huntington disease is suggested by the constellation of symptoms and a positive family history. Neuroimaging demonstrates atrophy of the basal ganglion structures (putamen and caudate). Genetic testing is clinically available and performed by measuring the repeat size in the *HD* gene, which can be accurately quantified by PCR. Presymptomatic testing for Huntington disease must be approached with great care because of the implications of a positive test for the patient and family. There is general consensus that asymptomatic children under the age of 18 years should never be tested. Until effective therapies are developed, all presymptomatic testing should be done with appropriate pre- and post-testing medical and psychological support services.

Progress towards therapy

Several transgenic mouse models for Huntington disease are proving useful in elucidating the mechanisms of the disease. A variety of agents are being administered to these genetically altered mice, as well as to human patients, in an attempt to slow the natural progression of the disorder by altering huntingtin protein aggregation, apoptosis or mitochondrial oxidation.

Myotonic dystrophy, type 1

Clinical features

Myotonic dystrophy, type 1, is a relatively common (~1/8000) neuromuscular autosomal dominant disorder with a highly variable phenotype. In the classic adult form, there is progressive muscle weakness along with continued contraction of muscles after cessation of voluntary effort (myotonia). Additional findings include cataracts, frontal baldness, disturbance of cardiac conduction and endocrine abnormalities. A milder adult form exists consisting of myotonia and cataracts. The most severe form is congenital myotonic dystrophy, in which infants are born with severe hypotonia, weakness and respiratory distress. Mental retardation is common among survivors. The number of trinucleotide repeats predicts the severity of the disease, and anticipation (*see* Chapter 2, p 55) is characteristic.

Gene and disease-related gene product

There is expansion of a CTG repeat in the 3′ untranslated region of the myotonia-dystrophica protein kinase gene, *DMPK* (19q13.3). The trinucleotide repeat is transcribed into mRNA but is not translated into the protein product. The mRNA containing the expanded triplet repeat appears to interfere with splicing of message encoding proteins, such as the muscle chloride channel, Clc-1, and cardiac troponin, which are required for normal muscle function.

Diagnosis

Findings on EMG and muscle biopsy are highly suggestive of myotonic dystrophy. A definitive diagnosis can be established by PCR or Southern blotting of the *DMPK* gene to determine the repeat size. This testing is widely available.

Progress towards therapy

Treatment is supportive. Identification of the mechanism underlying the disorder will increase our understanding of the disease and may pave the way for therapies.

Non mutation (Epigenetic) disorders

Description

Reversible alterations in the pattern of gene expression underlie a variety of disorders. Epigenetic disorders do *not* result from changes in the DNA

structure itself, but rather from abnormal gene expression caused by DNA methylation or chromatin modification (Chapter 2).

> **Epigenetics**
>
> Epigenetic modification can change the phenotype without changing the genotype.

Certain epigenetic modifications are normal, such as inactivation of one X chromosome in each female cell, or the silencing of certain genes depending on whether they are maternally or paternally inherited (so-called imprinted genes). Early proof that genes behaved differently depending on the gender of the parent from which they were inherited came from two naturally occurring tumours. Complete hydatidiform molar pregnancy is an abnormal conception with abnormal placental components but limited or non-existent development of the foetus. These molar pregnancies almost always possess a normal female chromosome complement (46, XX), but all the chromosomes derived from the father. Ovarian teratomas are sporadically occurring germ cell tumours that contain foetal elements, but little or no placental components. These tumours are also chromosomally normal female (46, XX) but all the chromosomes are maternal in origin. These findings demonstrated that simply having the correct chromosome and gene number was not sufficient to sustain normal development, but that inheritance of one gene copy from each parent was critical as well. In other words, some genes functioned differently (e.g. were imprinted) whether they were maternally or paternally inherited. To date, ~50 genes which undergo normal imprinting have been identified. *Imprinting* is a reversible event that occurs during gametogenesis; a gene that is normally imprinted or silenced during oogenesis, will be unimprinted during spermatogenesis.

Mutations that interfere with normal epigenetic modifications cause several human malformation syndromes. Several types of cancers are associated with epigenetic modifications that either silence tumour suppressor genes or activate tumour promoting genes. Hereditary nonpolyposis colorectal cancer is an example of this and is discussed on p 133.

Diagnosis

Diagnosis is disorder-specific, but can be made either by detection of abnormal methylation patterns of the gene/genes in question or identification of a mutation in an imprinting control centre gene (e.g. a gene controlling methylation patterns of nearby genes).

Therapy

Treatment is generally supportive for the specific medical problems associated with the disorder but potential treatments include use of RNAi or inhibitors of DNA methylation, such as 5-azacytidine.

Prader–Willi syndrome

Clinical features

Young infants with Prader–Willi syndrome have severe hypotonia and difficulty feeding. However, between one to six years of age, hyperphagia (excessive eating) and obesity develop. Additional features include subtle facial dysmorphology, hypogonadism, short stature in adolescence and adulthood and varying degrees of cognitive impairment which range from learning disabilities to mental retardation. Most cases are sporadic, with a negligible sibling recurrence risk.

Gene and disease-related gene product

Prader–Willi syndrome is caused by loss of a group of genes located at chromosome 15q11.2–13. Although the specific gene or genes responsible for the condition have not yet been identified, it is clear that loss of the paternal copy of this region is causal. Normally, several genes mapping to 15q11.2–13 are expressed only from the paternally inherited chromosome 15, while the second copy of these genes is silenced (or imprinted) by methylation on the maternally inherited chromosome 15. Prader–Willi syndrome occurs when patients do *not* express the paternally inherited genes in this region, either due to a chromosome deletion, maternal uniparental

disomy (both chromosome 15's are inherited from the mother) or a mutation that silences their expression. Several genes that map to 15q11.2–13 have been identified. The *SNRPN* (small nuclear ribonucleoprotein N) gene is involved in mRNA splicing, is expressed only from the paternally inherited chromosome 15 and most likely plays a role in Prader–Willi syndrome pathogenesis. For additional details on genes in this region, see section on Angelman syndrome (below).

Diagnosis

A chromosome 15q11.2–13 deletion can be detected cytogenetically or by FISH in ~70% of Prader–Willi syndrome cases. However, the most accurate diagnostic test takes advantage of differential methylation of genes in the Prader–Willi syndrome region. Specifically, PCR with methylation sensitive primers distinguishes the non-methylated paternally inherited genes from the methylated maternally inherited. This type of methylation assay is widely available.

Progress towards therapy

Standard treatments include administration of growth hormone starting in childhood, which has a very beneficial effect in preventing obesity and improving linear growth. Additional therapies are supportive.

Angelman syndrome

Clinical features

Angelman syndrome is a neurodevelopmental disorder characterized by mental retardation, gait ataxia and/or jerky limb movements, and a distinctive pattern of behaviours including inappropriate bursts of laughter or excitability. Additional findings can include minor facial dysmorphology, sleep disturbance, seizures, abnormal EEG pattern, post-natal microcephaly and severe impairment of expressive speech.

Gene and disease-related gene product

A small percent of patients with Angelman syndrome have a visible chromosome deletion of chromosome 15q11.2–13 and ~70% have a deletion of this region detectable by FISH. This finding initially caused considerable confusion as deletion of the same interval causes Prader–Willi syndrome, yet the two conditions have very distinct phentotypes. The explanation rests in the fact that selected genes in this region are 'imprinted', that is, either active or silent depending on the parent of origin. Absence of paternally inherited and active genes, such as *SNRPN*, contribute to Prader–Willi syndrome, while deletion or mutation of the maternally inherited copy of the gene, *UBE3A*, results in Angelman syndrome. This gene codes for a protein involved in the ubiquitination of other protein, a marker tagging proteins for degradation. Expression of the *UBE3A* gene is imprinted only in the brain. In other words, both maternal and paternal copies of *UBE3A* are expressed in non-CNS tissues, but only the maternal copy is expressed in CNS cells. This is consistent with Angelman syndrome being a neurodevelopmental disorder.

Diagnosis

Approximately 70% of cases of Angelman syndrome are caused by deletion of *UBE3A* at 15q11.2–13 on the maternally inherited chromosome #15, which can be detected by FISH. About 7% of cases are caused by paternal disomy which can be detected by DNA polymorphisms demonstrating that both copies of chromosome 15, or at least the 15q11.2–13 region, are inherited from the father. Specific mutations that eliminate the normal imprinting pattern of *UBE3A* or mutations in the *UBE3A* gene, itself, can be detected by sequencing. However, similar to Prader-Willi syndrome, the initial diagnostic test of choice is methylation analysis of the Prader–Willi syndrome/Angelman syndrome critical region at chromosome 15q11.2–13. Chromosome 15q11.2–13 deletions and uniparental disomy are usually sporadic occurrences, so that the risk of having another child with Angelman syndrome is low. However, mutations in the *UBE3A* gene can be inherited.

Progress toward therapy

Treatment is supportive.

Beckwith–Wiedemann syndrome

Clinical features

The Beckwith–Wiedemann syndrome (BWS) is an overgrowth syndrome associated with an increased risk for developing embryonal tumours, such as Wilms tumour, hepatoblastoma and rhabdomyosarcoma. Tumours occur in up to 10% of BWS individuals, usually during childhood. Frequent physical findings of BWS include macrosomia (large body size), macroglossia (enlarged tongue), anterior abdominal wall defects such as omphalocoele or umbilical hernia, hemihypertrophy (enlargement of 1 side of the body) and distinctive ear pits/creases. Overgrowth occurs during childhood, while adult size is generally normal. Intelligence is also usually normal. Most cases are sporadic with a negative family history, but ~15% have a positive family history with the disorder most often transmitted from an affected mother.

Gene and disease-related gene product

The chromosome location for BWS is 11p15.5 and several different genetic changes result in the condition. These changes share a common mechanism: abnormal expression of imprinted genes in the 11p15.5 region, but discussion of imprinted genes in this region, such as *IGF2* and *H19*, is beyond the scope of this book. Genotype–phenotype patterns are emerging, in that some mutations appear to be more tumourigenic, while others are associated with an increased risk for hemihypertrophy or omphalocele.

Diagnosis

A small percent of BWS patients have a chromosome abnormality involving 11p15.5 detected by standard techniques; polymorphic DNA repeats can be used to test for the presence of paternal disomy for chromosome 11. However, the best available diagnostic test, which is commercially available, identifies abnormal methylation of genes in this critical region.

Treatment

Current management involves medical and surgical treatment of existing problems and screening for tumours during childhood. An abdominal ultrasound examination should be performed, to assess for Wilms tumour and hepatoblastoma, every three months until the child is out of the high-risk period for tumour development, at ~8 years of age. Screening for hepatoblastoma should also be done by checking blood alphafetoprotein (AFP) level every six weeks until the child is 4 years of age.

Do assisted reproductive technologies increase the risk of having a child with an epigenetic disorder?

Assisted reproductive technologies, such as *in vitro* fertilization, gamete intrafallopian transfer, intracytoplasmic sperm injection, may increase the risk for having a child with Angelman or Beckwith–Wiedemann syndrome. The putative mechanism is that some aspect of embryo manipulation, such as components of the culture media, interferes with the normal process of methylation, and ultimately imprinting. Additional research will be required to resolve this issue.

Mitochondrial disorders

Description

Mitochondria are unique cytoplasmic organelles vital for cellular energy production (*see* p 58, Chapter 2). Mutations in either the mitochondrial genome, the extrachromosomal ~16 500 base pair DNA unique to mitochondria, or in the nuclear genes that code for mitochondrial components, can result in a mitochondrial disease.

Abnormalities in the mitochondrial DNA (mtDNA) fall into several categories:
(a) large deletions or duplications; these typically arise *de novo* or sporadically;
(b) point mutations in genes coding for proteins or RNAs; these typically are inherited from a mutation-carrying mother.

Collectively, mitochondrial disorders are not rare and have been estimated to affect as many as 1/8000 persons. mtDNA is double stranded and has 37 genes (with no introns) that code for two rRNA, 22 tRNAs and 13 proteins. The majority of mitochondrial components, which number over 1000, are therefore coded for by genes residing in nuclear DNA, with subsequent import of the protein product into the mitochondria. The mutation rate in mtDNA is considerably higher than that of nuclear DNA, contributing to the high frequency of mitochondrial disorders. Almost all of a person's mtDNA is maternally inherited, deriving from the oocyte at the time of conception; it is possible that some paternal mitochondria from the tail of the spermatozoa also enters the conceptus. However, mtDNA aberrations that run in families are always transmitted through the maternal line (e.g. maternal inheritance). Mitochondrial disorders caused by mutations in the nuclear genome most often follow an autosomal recessive pattern of inheritance.

The most common symptoms involve organs that have high energy requirements for normal function, such as the heart, brain, eye and skeletal muscle. Although some mitochondrial diseases cause symptoms in the newborn period, many do not present until adulthood. One possible explanation for this delay is that cumulative exposure to oxygen radicals is needed to further compromise mitochondrial function. There remain many unanswered questions about mitochondrial disorders and the mutations that cause them, such as why the same disorder can be produced by two very different mutations, or why the same mutation can produce two very different phenotypes.

Diagnosis

Elevated blood and spinal fluid lactate are consistent with mitochondrial disorders, but this is a non-specific screening test with many false positive and false negative results. The most straightforward mitochondrial disorders to diagnose are those due to a deletion, duplication or point mutation in the mtDNA. Such testing is commercially available and can be done on mtDNA extracted from blood, though heteroplasmy (mixture of mutant and normal mtDNA) can complicate interpretation of findings (*see* Box, below).

Mitochondrial DNA Mutations and Heteroplasmy

Mitochondrial DNA has a mutation rate 10 times that of nuclear DNA. Mutations can arise during oxidative phosphorylation when reactive oxygen species are generated and are favoured by the absence of normal DNA repair mechanisms and protective histones.

Individuals with mitochondrial mutations often have a mixture of normal and mutated mitochondrial DNA (a situation known as mitochondrial DNA heteroplasmy). The proportion of mutated mitochondrial DNA may vary between different individuals with the same mother, between tissues, and over time.

A few of the nuclear genome mutations that produce mitochondrial disorders can also be confirmed by genetic testing. In the absence of genetic confirmation of a mutation, a muscle biopsy is the next diagnostic step. The biopsy is processed in a specialized biochemistry laboratory to determine the activity of the respiratory chain complexes, as well as in a pathology laboratory to look for myopathic changes characteristic of mitochondrial disorders (e.g. ragged red muscle fibres).

Therapy

Treatment is generally supportive. Many patients are treated with co-enzyme Q10, a co-factor for transfer of electrons from complexes I and II to complex III. Patients with abnormalities of respiratory chain complex I or II may benefit from riboflavin supplementation. Among patients with mtDNA heteroplasmy, strategies to augment the number of normal mitochondria, or prevent duplication of mutant mitochondria are under discussion. Existing animal models of mitochondrial disorders fail to accurately recapitulate human phenotypes.

Polygenic disorders

Polygenic disorders

The common disorders of adult life are multifactorial in origin resulting from the effects of multiple environmental and genetic factors. The interaction of these factors give rise to the so-called complex traits such as diabetes, hypertension and Alzheimer disease. These conditions are far more common than the Mendelian and non-Mendelian disorders discussed above, affecting many millions of people worldwide. The identification of genes responsible for polygenic disorders has proved to be challenging since the multiplicative effect of several or even many genes result in the phenotype. However, the benefits of elucidating underlying genetic defects of common diseases are enormous as this will improve phenotypic classification, allow therapeutics to be designed and developed with specific genetic defects in mind, and ultimately permit treatments to be individually tailored, selecting drugs according to genetic abnormalities.

Unravelling the genetics of polygenic disorders

The nature of these diseases inevitably makes their genetic analysis complex. Three principal strategies have been used to identify susceptibility genes in polygenic disorders.

1 Linkage analysis looks for the segregation of traits with genetic markers beyond that expected by chance in families, and is applied to affected siblings or relative pairs to increase the power of detection (p 145).

2 Genetic association studies may be either population based or family based. In population-based studies affected and unaffected individuals are drawn from the population, and the frequency with which certain alleles occur in each of these groups is tested for association with a disease. Family-based studies search for association by detecting significant over-transmission of a particular allele with the disease or condition. All association studies are performed using a subset of known single nucleotide polymorphisms (SNPs) (*see* p 145) and currently require large numbers of patients.

3 Candidate genes can be sequenced to look for mutations. Candidate genes are genes that are predicted to be involved in the development of a multifactorial disease. For example, the genes involved in lipid metabolism are important candidates in trying to understand the polygenic inheritance of cardiovascular disease.

Consideration of recent advances in the mapping of loci for Alzheimer disease, diabetes mellitus and hypertension highlights both the achievements, and the potential difficulties, in unravelling the complexities of polygenic diseases.

Alzheimer disease

Alzheimer disease (AD), the most common form of dementia, is estimated to affect 12 million persons worldwide. It shows age-dependent prevalence with symptoms occurring in as many as 1/4 to 1/2 of persons over 85 years of age. Affected individuals demonstrate memory loss and progressive cognitive deterioration; additional features can include confusion, agitation and hallucinations. MRI scanning demonstrates no pathology other than diffuse cortical atrophy. AD is diagnosed in the presence of typical clinical findings, plus the exclusion of other causes of dementia. In most cases, disease onset is after 65 years of age, though a minority of patients demonstrate pre-senile or early-onset AD with symptoms starting after 40–50 years of age. AD is characterized pathologically by degeneration of neurons in the brain, particularly affecting the cerebral cortex and hippocampus. Aβ amyloid peptide, which is a fragment from the large membrane bound beta-amyloid precursor protein, form extracellular deposits. Inside cells 'tangled' tau proteins can be found.

There is increasing recognition that genetic factors contribute to AD. AD often aggregates in families, that is, affects more than one individual in the family. In fact 25% of persons with late-onset AD have an affected relative. There is considerable concordance for AD among both monozygotic and dizygotic twins. Three genes have been identified in which autosomal dominant, highly penetrant mutations are associated with an early-onset familial form of Alzheimer disease. These are the amyloid precursor protein (*APP*) gene on chromosome 21, presenilin 1 (*PS1*) on

chromosome 14 and presenilin 2 (*PS2*) on chromosome 1. The *APP* gene codes for the precursor protein that is cleaved to form Aβ amyloid peptide, a major component of the brain deposits found in patients with AD. Mutations in the *APP* gene produce abnormal APP protein cleavage products that are neurotoxic. The *PS1* and *PS2* genes code for highly homologous presenilin proteins that play a role in processing the protein APP; mutations in these genes also lead to the formation of abnormal APP protein cleavage products that are neurotoxic. However, less than 2% of AD patients are thought to carry one of these highly penetrant autosomal dominant mutations. The far more common late-onset AD is likely to be a complex disorder caused by mutations or variations in several susceptibility genes. Inheritance of the E4 allele of the apolipoprotein E gene (*APOE, see* Cardiovascular disease, below) is a risk factor that leads to earlier onset of symptoms. Persons of European descent who are homozygous for the E4 allele have a 3–4 fold excess risk for developing AD, compared to non-E4 carriers. One study recently identified a polymorphism in the gene ubiquilin 1 (*UBQLN1*, 9q22) that increases alternative splicing of this gene in the brain. The *UBQLN1* protein product is involved in protein degradation, possibly that of presenilin 1 and 2. The identification of genes associated with AD has provoked a debate concerning the value of genetic testing for the condition. Commercial tests are available to look for mutations in the three genes associated with early-onset familial AD and for genotyping *APOE* alleles, but no interventions have been proven to prevent or delay the onset of AD. Current recommendations are that while testing for highly penetrant mutations such as *PS1* can be justified for adults with the appropriate family history, *APOE* testing to predict and/or diagnose AD is not recommended.

Cardiovascular disease

Unravelling the genetic effects predisposing to cardiovascular disease is even more complex. Although some monogenic disorders such as familial hypercholesterolaemia (p 95) and various forms of hypertrophic cardiomyopathy (p 118) predispose to cardiovascular disease, most adult-onset cardiovascular disease is not due to a single gene disorder. Polygenic disorders such as hypertension and lipid abnormalities, and environmental effects such as cigarette smoking, all contribute to the development of atherosclerosis. One of the best studied genetically determined risk factors for cardiovascular disease is apolipoprotein E. Apolipoprotein E is a constituent of various lipoproteins and plays an important role in the transport of cholesterol and other lipids between cells. The *APOE* gene is polymorphic with three alleles (epsilon 2, epsilon 3 and epsilon 4), which code for isoforms E2, E3 and E4 each with different binding affinities for the apo E receptors. The E4 allele is associated with increased cholesterol levels, whilst the E2 allele is associated with elevated triglyceride levels. Although some studies support the role of apo E polymorphism in development of cardiovascular disease, the risk remains small in comparison to the risk associated with smoking or obesity.

Diabetes mellitus

Type 1 diabetes (Insulin-dependent diabetes mellitus or IDDM) is an autoimmune disorder in which the insulin-producing beta cells of the pancreas are destroyed. It tends to occur in children and young adults and appears to be increasing in frequency worldwide. The identical twin of a type 1 diabetic patient has a 30–50% chance of developing the disease, while a sibling has a 15-fold excess risk of developing the disorder compared to a nonrelated individual. These findings indicate that both genetic and nongenetic factors are involved in disease pathogenesis.

Two chromosome regions have been established for type 1 diabetes: the HLA (*see* Box "Human leukocyte antigens") class II genes (designated *IDDM1*; 6p21) and the insulin gene region (*IDDM2*; 11p15). More than a dozen other loci (IDDM 3–18) have been identified by linkage analysis and additional genes have been implicated in association studies. Future studies may not replicate all these findings. Diabetes type 1 appears to be truly polygenic in origin with multiple different loci conferring risk of developing the disorder.

Type 2 diabetes (Non-insulin-dependent diabetes mellitus or NIDDM) generally occurs in middle or old age and is increasing in frequency, affecting >150 million people worldwide. It is characterized by a resistance in tissues to the actions of insulin that is not adequately compensated for by increased insulin production from the pancreas. Genetically and clinically it is a heterogeneous disorder, but susceptibility genes have been identified, such as calpain 10, and glucose transporter genes, *GLUT2* and *GLUT4*. The identification of 'diabetogenic' genes has been aided by studies of an early-onset form of type 2 diabetes known as maturity-onset diabetes of the young (MODY). MODY is autosomal dominant and mutations in six different genes

Human Leucocyte Antigens

Human leucocyte antigens (HLA) are a family of glycoproteins that are encoded by genes within the major histocompatibility complex (MHC) on the short arm of chromosome 6. There are three HLA class I molecules, known as HLA-A, HLA-B and HLA-C, that are expressed on the surface of all nucleated cells, and three HLA class II molecules, known as HLA-DR, HLA-DP and HLA-DQ, that are normally expressed on a much smaller subset of cells, particularly lymphocytes, although their expression on other cell types can be induced during immune reactions. The function of both classes of HLA molecules is to bind pieces of proteins (peptides) and display them on the cell surface where they can be recognized by circulating T lymphocytes. HLA class I molecules bind peptides derived from intracellular parasites, such as viruses, and present them to cytotoxic T cells, which kill virally infected cells. HLA class II molecules bind peptides derived from extracellular pathogens and present them to helper T cells, which aid B lymphocytes in producing antibodies.

The genes encoding HLA antigens are extremely polymorphic, meaning that a large number of different alleles exist for each gene. Thus the pattern of HLA molecules expressed, known as the HLA type, varies considerably between individuals. While this is probably important for the health of the population because of the broader resistance to pathogens, it makes organ transplantation much more difficult because the recipient mounts a strong immune response against any different HLA molecules expressed on the donor tissue. The extent to which the HLA type of the donor matches that of a potential recipient is an important determinant of the survival of the graft.

involved in aspects of insulin processing have been identified. For example, a defect in the insulin promoter factor 1 gene appears to cause of maturity-onset diabetes of the young (*MODY4*), and may also be a significant risk factor for the development of type 2 diabetes.

Good control of blood sugar levels in diabetic patients can be achieved through the variety of available hypoglycaemic agents as well as new delivery systems, such as insulin pumps for continuous insulin infusion. However, these are symptomatic treatments and great efforts are underway to develop curative treatments through gene therapy approaches, especially in type 1 diabetes. Successful transplantation of purified beta-pancreatic islet cells has already been achieved but sources of donor cells are scarce and transplant recipients require immune suppression. Use of embryonic or adult stem cells that can differentiate into a variety of cell types, including islet cells, is under investigation in diabetic mouse models. One strategy is to 'transdifferentiate' cells *in vitro*; in other words, convert non-beta-cells into beta-cells or pancreatic islets by varying the culture medium *in vitro*, and then re-infuse these cells back into the diabetic animal model.

Hypertension

Hypertension is a disease of enormous public health importance in industrialized countries, since it is a major risk factor for the development of cardiovascular disease. Recent estimates are that 1.5 billion people worldwide will develop hypertension by the year 2025. The identification of susceptibility loci in 'idiopathic' or typical adult-onset hypertension has proven elusive. Blood pressure levels show strong familial aggregation which cannot be accounted for by shared environment alone. An individual is about twice as likely to develop hypertension if they have a hypertensive sibling. Several monogenic forms of hypertension have been identified, but in the majority of patients diverse genetic and environmental factors contribute to the condition. Understanding the physiological mechanisms involved in blood pressure control provides a basis for discovering responsible genes.

Monogenic (Mendelian) forms of hypertension:

1 Liddle's syndrome is an autosomal dominant disorder caused by a defect in either the beta or gamma subunits of a sodium channel found in epithelial cells. Premature truncation of either subunit (different pedigrees exist) causes constitutive activation of the channel, increasing sodium reabsorption by the tubules of the kidney. The result is salt-sensitive hypertension, associated with low plasma potassium and low levels of renin and aldosterone.

2 Apparent mineralocorticoid excess results from mutations in the gene encoding the enzyme 11beta-hydroxysteroid dehydrogenase, which is involved in conversion of the steroid cortisol to cortisone. While cortisol interacts with the mineralocorticoid receptor with a similar affinity to aldosterone, the affinity for cortisone is much lower. However, when the 11beta-hydroxysteroid dehydrogenase enzyme is deficient, normal circulating levels of cortisol can produce a marked mineralocorticoid effect. The result is early-onset hypertension with the features of mineralocorticoid excess, but very low plasma aldosterone levels.

3 In glucocorticoid-remediable aldosteronism, hypertension is associated with excessive secretion of aldosterone which is under the control of adrenocorticotrophic hormone (ACTH) rather than angiotensin II. Unequal crossing over during meiosis of the genes for 11 beta-hydroxylase and aldosterone synthase, which are close to each other on chromosome 8, produces a novel chimeric gene which is regulated by ACTH as if it were a cortisol-synthesizing gene.

Essential hypertension

These monogenic causes of hypertension are fascinating experiments of nature, but very rare. It is unclear to what extent mutations in these, and other genes which influence blood pressure, may contribute to the development of high blood pressure in the general population. For example, the renin angiotensin system plays a key role in blood pressure regulation, and genes encoding

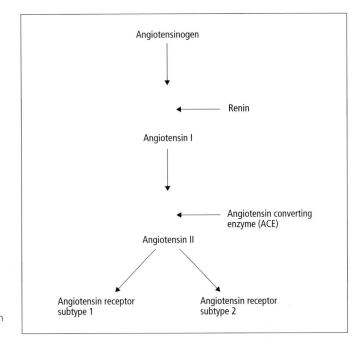

Figure 3.3 The renin angiotensin system.

components of the renin angiotensin system (Figure 3.3) have been studied extensively, but consistent associations with essential hypertension have been hard to identify.

Variations in the gene for angiotensinogen, which forms the substrate for renin, have been linked to hypertension in several European and Japanese studies, but not in African Americans. Angiotensin converting enzyme (ACE) converts angiotensin I to the potent vasoconstrictor angiotensin II. ACE is a highly polymorphic gene, and one of the most common variations is a deletion/insertion (D/I) of an Alu repeat (*see* p 60) in intron 16. The D allele has been associated with increased serum ACE activity, but reports of an association with essential hypertension have not been confirmed in large meta-analyses in which the results of many studies are combined. Angiotensin receptor subtype 1 mediates a number of the effects of angiotensin II, including vasoconstriction, vascular hypertrophy, left ventricular contractility and release of the hormone aldosterone, which promotes sodium retention by the kidney. Angiotensin receptor subtype 1 variants

have been associated with hypertension in a Finnish study, but no association was observed in African Americans.

The roles of other genes, including the epithelial sodium channel, components of the sympathetic nervous system, G-protein receptor subunits, regulators of vasoactive peptides such as endothelial nitric oxide synthase and alpha-adducin, the products of all of which would be expected to influence blood pressure, remain unclear.

Alpha-adducin in Human Hypertension

A mutation in the cell membrane associated protein alpha-adducin has recently been identified as the cause of high blood pressure in a spontaneously hypertensive strain of rat. Alpha-adducin may influence human blood pressure by regulating sodium reabsorption in the proximal tubule of the kidney, and a genetic variant, in which tryptophan replaces glycine as the 460th amino acid, has been associated with salt-sensitive hypertension. Carriers of the Trp460 variant experience a reduced risk of stroke or myocardial infarction if treated with thiazide diuretics, which inhibit sodium reabsorption in the distal tubule of the kidney, but not when treated with other antihypertensives.

Inconsistent findings related to the genetics of hypertension might arise from the inadequate power of small studies, variable susceptibility in different populations, varying interactions between genetic and environmental factors, and the combined effects of several disease-predisposing genetic variants. The challenges involved in identifying the genetic factors that contribute to variation in blood pressure highlight the challenges of dissecting the genetics of polygenic or multifactorial traits, but eventually knowledge of genetic variants that influence blood pressure may allow individualized tailoring of anti-hypertensive therapy.

Cancer – a multistep genetic disease

Cancers arise from the accumulation of genetic changes or mutations that cause growing cells to undergo malignant transformation. There are two broad families of cancer-causing genes, oncogenes and tumour suppressor genes; mutations in gene members of both families provides evidence that cancer has a genetic basis. Over 250 genes, or ~1% of the genes in the human genome, appear to play a role in the development of tumours.

Oncogenes

Retroviruses transcribe their RNA genome into DNA, which then becomes inserted into the host genome (p 143). Certain retroviruses contain genes which are capable of inducing malignant transformation in cells and can cause tumours in animals. These genes are called *viral oncogenes* or *v-onc* genes. DNA sequences that are homologous to *v-onc* genes are normally found in the genome of all vertebrate species. Thus almost all viral oncogenes have a normal cellular counterpart in the human genome, that is known as a cellular oncogene (*c-onc* gene) or proto-oncogene. Oncogenes are therefore evolutionarily conserved cellular genes encoding for proteins which have important regulatory functions in normal cell division and differentiation. However, oncogenes can be abnormally activated by chromosome rearrangements or point mutations and become

part of the mutation cascade that will transform a cell to malignancy.

Tumour suppressor genes

A second group of genes involved in the development of cancer are tumour suppressor genes, or anti-oncogenes. The presence of these genes in normal cells is thought to inhibit tumour development. Inactivating mutations in tumour suppressor genes result in loss of inhibition of cell cycle control favouring malignant transformation. Examples are the *p53* gene and the retinoblastoma gene (*see* p 139). The *p53* gene, on the short arm of chromosome 17, codes for a protein of the same name which is a transcription factor that can activate a wide range of genes involved in cell cycle arrest, induction of apoptosis and DNA repair. The cellular level of p53 protein increases dramatically in response to agents that damage DNA. One mechanism by which p53 regulates cell proliferation is that it induces another protein, p21, which is a cyclin-dependent kinase inhibitor that promotes growth arrest.

Normal *p53* function can be disrupted by mutation, althogh in some cases the *p53* gene is still intact but the p53 protein is inactivated. For example, the human papillomavirus E6 oncoprotein, a viral encoded transforming protein, binds to p53 and promotes its degradation. In ataxia telangiectasia an inherited defect leads to defective post-translational modification of p53 (*see* p 134).

How do mutations in these genes cause cancer?

Cancer develops when mutations disrupt the normal function of oncogenes or tumour suppressor genes in regulating cell growth, proliferation and death. This can occur in a number of ways. Inactivation of tumour suppressor function by gene deletion or abnormal epigenetic modification (*see* p 123) can disrupt cell cycle control checkpoints. Mutations in an oncogene may activate it, leading to production of an abnormal protein product. Oncogene expression may be increased by amplification, occuring when the gene is present in multiple copies. Chromosome breakage involved in translocations may disrupt the oncogene or bring it under the control of different promoter regions. A number of consistent chromosomal translocations have been described in human malignancies, leading to the identification of an oncogene at the breakpoint.

Familial versus sporadic cancers

In ~10% of cancers the primary tumour-promoting mutation is inherited while the remaining 90% of cancers are caused by accumulation of somatic or acquired mutations (*see* Box "Germline versus somatic mutations", p 132).

Familial cancers

Most familial cancers involve inactivation of tumour suppressor genes. Loss of function of *both* copies of the gene, or so-called two hits, is onco-

genic. In familial cancers one functioning copy of the gene is lost in the germline (either inherited from an affected parent or arising as a new mutation in the sperm or the egg). Thus, at the time of birth every cell in the body already has one-hit, that is, one non-functioning copy of the gene. Loss of the second copy of the gene, or the second hit, is acquired by mutation, deletion or epigenetic modification (*see* Figure 3.4 – Knudson's two-hit hypothesis; also see Retinoblastoma, p 139). Sporadic cancers that are due to inactivation of tumour suppressor genes must acquire both hits independently after birth. Accordingly, the risk for tumour development is far greater in familial cancers and these are likely to have an earlier onset and be multifocal compared to their sporadic counterparts. Understanding the disease mechanisms underlying familial cancers provides valuable insights into the role of these genes.

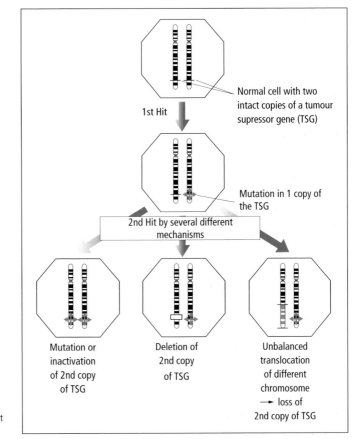

Figure 3.4 Knudson's 2 hit hypothesis.

Germline Versus Somatic Mutations

A mutation present in a germ cell (e.g. egg or sperm) that can be passed to offspring where it will be present in every cell in the body. A somatic mutation arises in a single cell post-conception and is passed on only to the progeny of that cell. Unless these progeny include a germ cell, somatic mutations cannot be passed on to the offspring of the individual.

Ataxia telangiectasia

Clinical features

An autosomal recessive childhood-onset disorder characterized by progressive loss of coordination (cerebellar ataxia) and dilatation of small blood vessels, particularly in the eye (ocular telangiectasia). Patients also suffer from immunodeficiency, chromosomal instability, hypersensitivity to ionizing radiation and a predisposition to cancer, especially leukaemias and lymphomas. For a person with ataxia telangiectasia, the lifetime risk of developing some form of cancer approaches 40%. Heterozygote carriers of an *ATM* mutation are at an increased risk for developing breast cancer.

Gene and disease-related gene product

Ataxia telangiectasia is one of several 'genetic instability' syndromes, all of which are caused by mutations in DNA damage repair systems. The product of the *ATM* (ataxia telangiectasia mutated) gene (11q22.3) is vital for repairing double-stranded DNA breaks. It is a kinase that is required for the normal function of other genes such as *p53* (p 132); mutations in *ATM* disrupt cell cycle control as well as DNA repair. Over 400 mutations have been found in *ATM*, so most families have private mutations. The protein product is widely expressed but is most abundant in the affected organs, namely the brain, thymus and spleen.

Diagnosis

Elevated blood levels of alphafetoprotein suggest the diagnosis and are found in ~90% of patients.

Additional supportive findings include breaks and rearrangements on routine chromosome analysis (especially a translocation between chromosomes 7 and 14), recurrent infections, decreased immunoglobulin levels and telangiectasias. The diagnosis is confirmed by either detecting the mutant protein (using a protein truncation assay) or by genetic testing which is clinically available. The latter is performed by either directed mutation screening or by sequencing the entire *ATM* gene, with >90% detection rate.

Progress towards therapy

Molecular analysis of the disorder has provided valuable insights into the cellular response and cancer risk associated with radiation exposure. No specific therapy to ameliorate the course of this disorder currently exists.

Breast cancer

Clinical features

Approximately 5–10% of all cases of breast cancer are hereditary due to a mutation in a single gene. The most common form of hereditary breast cancer results from inheritance of highly penetrant dominant mutations in the genes *BRCA1* and *BRCA2*. In high risk groups, such as women of Ashkenazi Jewish descent or families with two cases of young onset breast cancer, at least 20% of cases are attributable to *BRCA1* or *BRCA2* mutations. Among mutation carriers, penetrance for breast cancer is high, with as many as 80% of women developing breast cancer in their lifetime. The penetrance for ovarian cancer is somewhat lower but as many as 50–60% have a lifetime risk of developing ovarian cancer. The likelihood of developing cancer appears to be lower in non-Ashkenazi Jewish mutation carriers. Up to 15% of male breast cancer cases are due to a mutation in *BRCA2*. Other cancers, such as prostate and pancreatic, are more common among mutation carriers.

Since a substantial percentage of breast cancer families do *not* demonstrate a *BRCA1* or *BRCA2* mutation, searches for additional genes that predispose to breast cancer are underway.

Gene and disease-related gene product

BRCA1 and *BRCA2* have complex structures without homology to other known genes. They both code for nuclear proteins and *BRCA1* plays important roles in DNA-damage response pathways, cell cycle control and development. The *BRCA1* gene (17q21) encodes a nuclear protein of 1863 amino acids that contains a RING finger domain, and a tandemly repeated BRCA1C-terminal domain thought to be involved in cell cycle regulation. *BRCA1* interacts with the protein Rad51, which has been identified in yeast as a major regulator of DNA repair and recombination. *BRCA2* (13q12.3) can interact with Rad51 and has domains that can act as transcriptional regulators.

Mutations in these genes generally result in protein truncation and as predicted by Knudson's two-hit model, loss of the second copy of the gene promotes tumour development.

Diagnosis

Three common changes account for 90% of *BRCA1* and *BRCA2* mutations among women of Ashkenazi Jewish descent. Targeted mutation analysis for this ethnic group is widely available. Among women of all ethnic groups who demonstrate linkage to either the *BRCA1* or *BRCA2* locus, complete gene sequencing will detect mutations in approximately 90%. Gene sequencing is also commercially available. Genetic testing will allow reassurance for women who have not inherited a mutated gene. Although identification of mutation carriers may raise psychological stress for the patient, there is now evidence that appropriate prophylactic treatment, such as mastectomy and/or oophorectomy, can reduce the risk of developing cancer.

Ring Finger

The RING finger motif is a specialized zinc finger domain (*see* Box, "Transcription and Control Regions", p 19) found in many transcriptional regulatory proteins.

Colon cancer

Five to ten percent of colon cancers follow an autosomal dominant pattern of inheritance, and the two major forms of colorectal cancer in which high penetrance genetic mutations have been identified are hereditary nonpolyposis colorectal cancer (HNPCC) and familial adenomatosis polyposis (FAP). The contribution from low penetrance mutations to the pathogenesis of most of the remaining cases of familial colorectal cancer is unknown. Extensive research into the role of genetic and environmental factors, and in particular diet, is ongoing.

Lifestyle and diet in risk of colon cancer

Physical inactivity and excess body weight, particularly a central deposition of fat, and smoking early in life, are consistent risk factors for colon cancer. Diets high in red and processed meat, and perhaps refined carbohydrates, also increase risk. Excess alcohol consumption, probably in combination with a diet low in nutrients such as folic acid, appears to increase risk, while calcium and vitamin D may be protective. The relationship between dietary fibre and risk of colon cancer remains controversial.

Familial adenomatous polyposis

Clinical features

Familial adenomatous polyposis (FAP) is a hereditary form of colorectal cancer in which affected individuals develop numerous adenomatous polyps of the large intestine. In classic FAP, mean age of polyp onset is 16 years and by age 35, all affected individuals have hundreds to thousands of polyps. Ultimately, one or more of the polyps undergoes malignant transformation so that 100% of untreated individuals develop colon cancer by age 40. Endoscopic screening for polyps should begin by age 10. Treatment to prevent colon cancer consists of prophylactic proctocolectomy (surgical removal of colon and rectum) once adenomas are present. Additional extra-colonic manifestations can occur including: osteomas and soft tissue tumours (a constellation referred to as Gardner syndrome), as well as congenital hypertrophy of the retinal pigment epithelium, dental abnormalities and non-colonic malignancies. In a milder form of the disorder, so-called attenuated FAP, less than 100 colonic polyps are present; malignant transformation of polyps occurs at a later age.

Gene and disease-related gene product

The most common form of FAP is an autosomal dominant disorder due to mutations in the adenomatosis polyposis coli (APC) gene at 5q21. APC codes for a tumour suppressor protein that controls cell proliferation by acting on the *WNT* signalling pathway and down-regulating the expression of *c-MYC*, an oncogene. Some specific genotype–phenotype correlations are noted; for instance, mutations in the 3' or 5' end of *APC* are associated with attenuated FAP. Among Ashkenazi Jews, a single base pair change in codon 1307 results in a long tract of adenines in the APC protein. This base pair change is present in ~6% Ashkenazi Jews and is associated with a doubling in the risk of colorectal cancer.

Diagnosis

Until discovery that mutations in *APC* were the cause of FAP, the diagnosis was made by detection of polyps on colonoscopy. Now, gene sequencing can identify an *APC* mutation in ~90% of affecteds. All first-degree relatives of a patient with a confirmed mutation must also be offered mutation screening. Mutation testing is commercially available. In 75% of cases FAP is inherited from an affected parent, while in 25% the family history is negative consistent with the presence of a *de novo APC* mutation in the affected individual.

Hereditary nonpolyposis colon cancer

Clinical features

HNPCC is an autosomal dominant syndrome of bowel cancer that accounts for up to 5% of all colorectal cancer diagnoses. It results from germline mutations in mismatch repair (MMR) genes. Among the hereditary colon cancers, HNPCC is more common than FAP. Individuals with HNPCC have an 80% risk of colorectal cancer by age 70, and tumours most often occur in the proximal colon. In contrast to FAP, HNPCC is not associated with a massively increased number of adenomatous colorectal polyps. However, polyps are more likely to form at an earlier age and become malignant compared to persons in the general population. Since HNPCC is not characterized by a profusion of polyps there is no clinical phenotype until a cancer develops. There is also an increased risk of cancer at a variety of sites. Almost half of females develop cancer of the endometrium; other common sites of malignancy involve the ovary, stomach, small bowel, hepatobiliary tract and urinary tract.

Gene and disease-related gene product

Mismatch repair involves the recognition and correction of complementary base pair errors; specifically, repair occurs when a normal nucleotide sequence on one strand of DNA is either unpaired or incorrectly matched with a base pair on the complementary strand. Mutations in the genes human mutS homologue 2 (*hMSH2*, 2p22–p21) and human mutL (*E. coli*) homologue 1 (*hMLH1*; 3p21.3) are found in the majority of HNPCC families. The protein product of *hMSH2* can pair with one of two other mismatch repair proteins, hMSH6 or hMSH3, and the dimeric protein complex recognizes errors that may have occurred during DNA replication. The hMLH1 protein product is another component of the DNA mismatch repair pathway, which can form a heterodimer with hMLH3, hPMS2 or hPMS1 and may interact with hMSH2 to recruit enzymes, including helicase, exonucle-ase and polymerase, to repair the error. One of the consequence of a mutation in a MMR gene is that stretches of repetitive DNA, known as microsatellite regions, can expand or contract, a phenomenon referred to as microsatellite insta-bility (MSI). More than 90% of colorectal carci-noma patients with mutations in *hMSH2* or *hMLH1* demonstrate a high-frequency of MSI in tumour samples.

Diagnosis

Testing for HNPCC is complex because several genes are involved, with a total of more than 400 known mutations. Staining of tumour samples for the presence of the MLH1 or MSH2 proteins or analysis of genetic material from tumours for MSI can be used to select patients for HNPCC mutation testing. Expert committees have devel-oped diagnostic criteria, such as the *Bethesda cri-teria*, to determine whether a person with colorectal cancers should have their tumour tested for MSI. Several important features of these criteria are:

1 HNPCC-related cancers or associated extra-colonic cancers;

2 colorectal cancer and a first-degree relative with colorectal cancer and/or HNPCC-related extra-colonic cancer and/or a colorectal adenoma; one of the cancers diagnosed at age <45 years, and the adenoma diagnosed at age <40 years;

3 colorectal cancer or endometrial cancer diag-nosed at age <50 years;

4 right-sided colorectal cancer with an undiffer-entiated pattern on histopathology diagnosed at age <45 years;

5 Individuals with signet ring cell type colorectal cancer diagnosed at age <45 years;

6 Individuals with adenomas diagnosed at age <40 years.

The identification of individuals with an HNPCC mutation allows screening of at-risk fam-ily members, who can then be included in special surveillance programmes, using tests such as regu-lar colonoscopy.

Li–Fraumeni syndrome

Clinical features

In Li–Fraumeni syndrome inheritance of only one functional copy of the *p53* gene (*see* p 130) predisposes to the early development of several diverse cancers, which are clinically and histopathologically indistinguishable from their counterparts that arise in the general population. Approximately 50% of cancers in individuals with Li–Fraumeni syndrome occur before 30 years of age. Adrenocortical tumours occur in infancy, soft tissue sarcomas in the first 5 years of life and osteosarcomas in adolescence. Acute leukaemia and brain tumours also occur throughout childhood and young adulthood. Premenopausal breast cancer is the commonest cancer in young adults. Cancer patients in these families who survive their first neoplasm are prone to develop second cancers, particularly within the field of radiation therapy.

Gene and disease-related gene product

p53 (17p13.1) codes for a transcription factor that activates expression of a large number of genes which are thought to prevent accumula-tion of DNA mutations in cells. Although Li–Fraumeni syndrome is rare, mutations in *p53* can be found in many sporadic human malignan-cies; these mutations, 'acquired' during the life-time of the cell, emphasize the importance of this gene in protecting against the development of cancer.

Diagnosis

The clinical diagnosis is based on the aggregation of two or more of the cancers currently known to occur in the syndrome. Fewer than 400 families worldwide have been diagnosed with the condi-tion. Predictive testing for germline *p53* mutations is technically feasible, but the overall benefit of this is unclear.

Multiple endocrine neoplasia 1

Clinical features

An autosomal dominant disorder in which benign and malignant tumours arise in endocrine organs. The most common manifestations include hyperparathyroidism secondary to parathyroid adenoma, duodenal gastrointestinal tumours, pancreatic tumours and anterior pituitary tumours. Half of the patients develop symptoms of either hormone excess or tumours by age 20 and all manifest symptoms by 50 years of age. Approximately one-third of patients die from disease-related malignances.

Gene and disease-related gene product

Defects occur in the gene *MEN-1* (multiple endocrine neoplasia 1) (11q13) encoding the menin protein. The function of menin is as yet unknown but it interacts with a number of proteins that play a role in regulating cell growth; accordingly, mutations in menin allow unregulated cell growth resulting in malignancy.

Diagnosis

A mutation in *MEN-1* can be found in 80–90% of patients. There are no mutation hot spots but as predicted by Knudson's two-hit hypothesis (Fig 3.4), most are loss-of-function mutations resulting in diminished or absent activity of the protein product. *MEN-1* mutation testing is available in selected DNA diagnostic laboratories. Establishing the diagnosis allows for appropriate medical management; prophylactic surgery, especially involving the pancreas and duodenum is controversial. First-degree relatives of a confirmed case of MEN-1 should undergo genetic testing to determine whether or not they carry the same disease-causing mutation.

Neurofibromatosis

Neurofibromatosis was first described in 1882 by Dr Friedrich von Recklinghausen. The most common form is neurofibromatosis type I (NF 1).

Neurofibromatosis type 1 (von Recklinghausen disease)

Clinical features

A very common autosomal dominant disorder affecting 1 in 3000 persons. The condition is diagnosed by the presence of at least two of the following: six or more pigmented skin lesions (café au lait spots) >15 mm in size in adults, freckling in the axillae and/or inguinal regions, two or more neurofibromas, optic glioma (tumour of the optic nerve or chiasm), two or more Lisch nodules (benign hamartomas of the iris of the eye) or a first-degree relative with NF1. The most common type of tumour is the cutaneous or dermal neurofibroma. These are discrete benign growths along nerve sheaths, consisting of a mixture of cells including Schwann cells and fibroblasts. These small neurofibromas can accumulate over time, can number in the dozens or hundreds scattered over the body, but rarely convert to a malignant form. A less common type of neurofibroma, the plexiform neurofibroma, is a congenital tumour involving multiple nerve roots or bundles that can transform to a malignant state. Other features that have been reported include macrocephaly, scoliosis, pheochromocytoma (a tumour of the adrenal gland), learning disabilities and hypertension. Café au lait spots are often present at birth or appear during infancy, while additional NF1 manifestations appear during childhood and adolescence. The lifetime risk that a person with NF1 develops a malignancy is ~5%.

Gene and disease-related gene product

Part of the protein, neurofibromin, encoded by *NF1* (17q11) is similar to the GTPase activating protein family and down-regulates the activity of RAS, a key molecular signal for many cellular functions. However, the exact function of neurofibromin is not yet fully understood. Over 80% of germline mutations predict severe truncation of the neurofibromin protein.

Diagnosis

Although DNA-based testing, as well as a neurofibromin protein truncation assay are available, they are rarely used for diagnosis. The diagnosis is still established clinically by meeting the criteria presented above. About half of patients with NF1 inherit the disorder from an affected parent while the disorder arises as a *de novo* or new dominant mutation in the remainder.

Neurofibromatosis type 2

Clinical features

An autosomal dominant disorder occurring in 1 in 40 000 persons that is characterized by bilateral benign tumours of the nervous system, containing Schwann cells, glial cells and meningeal cells. The most common tumours involve the auditory nerves and are designated vestibular schwannomas. Additional tumours such as schwannomas of other nerves, meningiomas and gliomas can occur. Vestibular Schwannomas are present in affected persons by age 30 years. Hearing loss beginning in the teens or early adult life is usually the first symptom, but other symptoms referable to the VIIIth cranial nerve, such as tinnitus or balance problems, are common as well. A variety of other central and peripheral nervous tumours can also occur.

Gene and disease-related gene product

The neurofibromatosis 2 (*NF2*; 22q12.2) gene product has been named merlin, for *m*oezin-*e*zrin*r*adixin *li*ke protei*n*, because of its similarity to these cytoskeletal proteins. Merlin interacts with numerous other proteins and plays a role in the Ras/Rac pathway. *NF2* probably acts as a tumour suppressor gene so that loss of both copies of the gene promotes tumourogenesis.

Diagnosis

The diagnosis is established using clinical criteria. DNA-based mutation analysis is available clinically for confirmation of the diagnosis and for early detection of at-risk individuals (usually children of affected patients). Approximately half the cases of NF2 are caused by a *de novo* or new dominant mutation.

Retinoblastoma

Clinical features

Retinoblastoma is a malignant tumour of the retina affecting about 1 in 20 000 children. Both hereditary and non-hereditary forms exist. In the 10% of cases where the mutation is inherited (i.e. present in the affected patient's germline) multiple tumours are generally found in both eyes and develop within the first 5 years of life. The presence of a single tumour in one eye is more common in the non-hereditary form, but does not exclude the hereditary form since some mutations have low penetrance. As more children have become long-term survivors, it is apparent that they are at increased risk for developing osteosarcoma and other tumours in later life. Approximately 25% of retinoblastoma survivors develop a second cancer and the risk is greatest for those who received radiation therapy.

Gene and disease-related gene product

The retinoblastoma 1 gene (*RB1*, 13q14.2) codes for the retinoblastoma 1 protein which is thought to act as a negative regulator of cell proliferation by sequestering nuclear proteins involved in cell growth. Knudson postulated his two-hit hypothesis for tumour suppressor genes based on findings in retinoblastoma (Figure 3.4). Familial cases are dominantly inherited. In retinoblastoma families, a mutation in *RB1* is inherited on one chromosome 13 (e.g. the first hit) and is present in all cells in the body; when a retinal cell suffers a sporadic mutation, deletion or translocation which inactivates the second copy of *RB1* (e.g. the second hit) this cell is likely to become malignant resulting in a retinal tumour. Sporadic cases require two separate and *de novo* hits, one to inactivate each copy of *RB1*.

Diagnosis

The most common presenting symptoms are loss of the normal red reflex (replaced by a white reflex known as leukocoria) and strabismus (lazy eye). Examination of the back of the eye using an ophthalmoscope reveals the tumour. Untreated, retinoblastoma is almost uniformly fatal, but with early diagnosis and modern methods of treatment the survival rate is over 90%. Treatment options include radiotherapy, light coagulation (photocoagulation), cryotherapy and thermotherapy delivered by infrared radiation. Standard chromosome analysis should be performed on all patients with retinoblastoma as 5–8% will have a deletion involving 13q14; additional problems such as birth defects and/or mental retardations are found in these patients. Most individuals with retinoblastoma have a point mutation, small deletion or hypermethylation in *RB1*; testing for these abnormalities is commercially available in specialized DNA diagnostic laboratories using techniques such as FISH, targeted PCR, full gene sequencing or comparison of patterns of polymorphic markers between parents and the affected child (to identify loss of heterozygosity). Molecular testing to confirm the presence and type of *RB1* mutation in the proband is a key component in the management of retinoblastoma. This must be accompanied by genetic counselling for interpretation of molecular studies, to identify other at-risk family members, and to assess whether molecular testing of them is indicated. Screening protocols for detecting second tumours is also a vital part of the long-term management of a patient with retinoblastoma.

Tuberous sclerosis complex, types 1 and 2

Clinical features

An autosomal dominant condition affecting about 1 in 6000 children in which multiple benign tumours known as hamartomata commonly occur in the skin, retina, brain and kidneys. Criteria from the Tuberous Sclerosis Complex Consensus Conference were published in 1998 and are used for clinical diagnosis of the disorder. These criteria consist of a combination of major and minor findings. Major findings include facial angiofibroma (formerly known as adenoma sebaceum), brain hamartomas (consisting of cortical tubers and subependymal nodules), cardiac rhabdomyoma and the presence of three or more hypopigmented spots (macules) on the skin. Some of the recognized minor criteria are pits of tooth enamel, renal cysts and gingival fibromas. Epilepsy, mental retardation and/or learning difficulties are often present. In the kidney benign tumours known as angiomyolipomata (hamartomas made up of vascular tissue (angio), smooth muscle (myo), and fat (lipoma)) often compress healthy renal tissue although they rarely cause renal failure.

Gene and disease-related gene products

The disease can be caused by mutations in either of two genes. *TSC1* (9q34) encodes the protein hamartin which has no clear homology to other vertebrate proteins. *TSC2* (16p13) encodes the protein tuberin which shows some homology to GTPase-activating proteins. Hamartin and tuberin associate *in vivo*, suggesting that they function in the same complex. They both appear to function as tumour suppressor genes. Two-thirds of patients diagnosed with tuberous sclerosis have a negative family history, indicating that the disorder most often arises as a new dominant mutation.

Diagnosis

Clinical diagnostic criteria, based on the presence of typical findings, have been devised. Genetic testing to detect mutations and deletions in both *TSC1* and *TSC2* confirms the diagnosis in up to 75% of patients and is commercially available. Parents should be carefully examined to determine whether one of them has physical evidence of tuberous sclerosis. Genetic testing should be performed on the index case. If a mutation is identified, then the proband's parents should also be tested to see if one of them has the mutation. Most mutations are private, e.g., are unique to each family.

Von Hippel–Lindau syndrome

Clinical features

An autosomal dominant condition characterized by the abnormal growth of capillary blood vessels leading to hemangioblastomas. Hemangioblastoma formation commonly occurs in the central nervous system, especially in the cerebellar hemispheres of the brain, and the retina. CNS lesions cause a variety of neurological abnormalities while retinal lesions may be asymptomatic or produce a visual field deficit. Renal carcinoma, which occurs in about 40% of affected individuals, is the leading cause of mortality. Sudden deafness can result from tumour involvement of the endolymphatic sac and duct of the membranous labyrinth of the internal ear.

Gene and disease-related gene product

The Von Hippel–Lindau disease tumour suppressor protein (pVHL) is coded for by the *VHL* gene (3p26). pVHL also forms part of a multi-protein complex involved in ubiquitination, a process that targets proteins for degradation. This complex specifically transfers ubiquitin onto the transcription factor, hypoxia inducible factor (HIF1α), targeting it for degradation. HIF1α regulates vascular endothelial growth factor (VEGF) expression, so that deficiency in pVHL leads to overexpression of VEGF, which in turn could contribute to hemangioblastoma formation.

Diagnosis

The diagnosis is suspected in individuals with typical lesions including hemangioblastomas and renal carcinoma, and can be confirmed by detection of mutations in *VHL*. Presymptomatic diagnosis is possible by DNA analysis, allowing surveillance for tumours. Over three-quarters of cases are familial though it may be difficult to identify the affected parent clinically due to incomplete penetrance or failure to recognize signs of the disease.

Wilms tumour

Clinical features

Wilms tumour is an embryonal malignancy of the kidney. It affects about 1 in 10 000 children and accounts for about 8% of childhood cancers. It is believed to result from malignant transformation of stem cells, which remain in the kidney beyond birth. 75% occur before the age of 5, and 2–5% are bilateral. Approximately 2% of affected children have a family history of Wilms tumour, and even sporadic Wilms tumour is thought to have a strong genetic component. Familial cases generally have an earlier age of onset and an increased frequency of bilateral disease.

Gene and disease-related gene product

One Wilms' tumour suppressor gene (*WT1*) (11p13) encodes a transcription factor that is critical to normal kidney and gonadal development. A second Wilms' tumour suppressor gene has been identified at 11p15, and linkage studies suggest that further loci may exist.

Diagnosis

The presence of Wilms tumour is usually established by ultrasound examination or CT scanning. The extent of spread and stage of the tumour determines the role of surgery, radiotherapy and chemotherapy in treatment.

Sporadic cancer

Most cancers are sporadic, in which new genetic mutations arise in cells rather than being inherited.

Chronic myeloid leukaemia – an example of a sporadic cancer

Chronic myeloid leukaemia (CML) results from the proliferation of abnormal white blood cell precursors in the bone marrow. It comprises ~10% of all adult leukaemias. In about 90% of patients there is an apparently balanced translocation (p 60) involving exchange of chromosomal material between chromosomes 9 and 22 in the malignant cells. This gives rise to a shortened chromosome 22 known as the Philadelphia chromosome. This chromosomal rearrangement results in the translocation of the *bcr* (breakpoint cluster region) gene (22q11) adjacent to the *c-abl* (abelson oncogene) gene (9q34) resulting in a fusion gene. The newly created fusion gene produces a BCR–ABL fusion protein that localizes to the cytoskeleton and displays continuous tyrosine kinase activity within cells.

Tyrosine kinases are enzymes that transfer phosphate groups from ATP to the hydroxyl group of tyrosine residues on molecules involved in signalling within cells. Tyrosine kinases control many fundamental processes of cells, such as cell proliferation, differentiation, motility, death or survival. In tumour cells tyrosine kinases escape normal regulation and sustain signal transduction pathways in an activated state. The drug imatinib mesylate (Gleevec) binds to the BCR–ABL fusion protein and neutralizes the tyrosine kinase activity. Imatinib blocks the growth of these leukaemia cells, and induces apoptosis. Clinical studies of imatinib have yielded impressive results in the treatment of CML. Since uncontrolled tyrosine kinases activity is common in tumour cells, small molecule inhibitors of tyrosine kinases such as imatinib are emerging as important therapeutic agents in cancer treatment.

Impact of molecular biology on cancer therapy

Hopes that genetic approaches would lead to advances in cancer therapy through development of cancer vaccines, in which tumour cells are manipulated to provoke an immune response, or gene therapy in which genetic manipulation is used to deliver specific therapies to cancer cells, have so far proved speculative. However, one of the major impacts of molecular biology on cancer diagnosis and treatment has been the molecular classification of cancer. Pathologists have traditionally relied on microscopic examination to classify tumours.

The identification of many genes involved in cancer could revolutionize the way in which tumours are classified. Classification according to genetic defects is likely to guide specific treatments and improve prediction of clinical outcome. In addition, molecular assessment of tumour margins and regional lymph nodes may improve staging of tumours. Studies applying techniques, such as DNA microarray and SAGE to simultaneously monitor expression of thousands of genes, are underway to provide a detailed basis of the molecular basis of tumour development and growth.

Gene therapy – promises and problems

The identification of the genetic defect underlying many diseases led to speculation that genetic disorders could be treated by gene therapy. Efforts have focused on somatic gene therapy, in which the function of mutated genes is corrected in specific cells or organs rather than in egg or sperm cells or early embryos (germline therapy). Two approaches have been used, *ex vivo* and *in vivo* gene delivery. In *ex vivo* delivery cells are taken from a patient, the new gene is inserted and the cells are then replaced back into the patient. *In vivo* delivery involves delivering the gene directly to the patient's tissues, usually by infecting them with a virus that contains the new gene.

Before considering the possibility of gene therapy:

- the gene must have been cloned and sequenced so that it is fully characterized and readily available in its correct form;
- it must be possible to introduce the gene safely and efficiently into appropriate target cells;
- the gene must then be expressed in its new site.

The commonest approach has been to incorporate the gene into a virus, which is then used to infect target cells. Viruses have evolved to incorporate nucleic acid into cells and induce new gene expression, often without cytotoxicity. They are thus ideally suited to achieve a high efficiency of gene transfer and expression. In modifying a virus so that it can safely deliver a new gene, endogenous harmful viral genes are removed; however, the potential risk that these engineered viruses (so-called viral vectors) may cause disease remains.

Viral delivery systems

Potential risks of viral vectors:
- Viral vectors which integrate into the genome may cause DNA mutations (insertional mutagenesis).
- Recombination of the disabled viral vector with wild-type virus may lead to infectious complications
- The virus can induce an inflammatory and immune response.

RNA viruses – retroviral vectors

RNA viruses are usually small (less than 20 kb). Many amplify and transcribe their genomes exclusively in the cytoplasm of mammalian cells, resulting in high levels of expression without the risks associated with integration into host cell DNA. Cytoplasmic expression is usually transient. This limits applications to short-term gene therapy, such as the treatment of cancer. Their role in vaccine development is also being explored.

Retroviruses have a single stranded RNA genome, which is converted into DNA by reverse transcriptase carried by the virus particle. The DNA is then incorporated into the host genome, where it is expressed to produce new viral RNA, together with proteins needed to form new viral particles. Retroviruses can be prepared for gene therapy by replacing some of the viral genes with the gene to be used for therapy. One of the major advantages of retroviruses is their high efficiency of integration into the host genome, which is followed by stable expression of the introduced gene

even after cell division. However, infection of non-replicating cells is poor, and the stability of the virus is adversely affected by the introduction of large gene inserts. Retroviruses are therefore best suited for the introduction of small genes into replicating cells.

Adenoviruses

Adenoviruses are double-stranded DNA viruses which have been used in live viral vaccines for many years, providing a long safety record. Adenoviruses can infect non-dividing cells, but viral DNA does not integrate efficiently into the host genome, and may not be transferred to daughter cells. This raises the possibility that in tissues undergoing cell turnover, introduced DNA may be lost and need to be reintroduced at regular intervals. Adenoviruses have been used in trials of gene therapy for respiratory disorders because of the tendency of the virus to infect cells lining the airways.

Herpes simplex virus type-1

HSV-1 (Herpes simplex virus type-1) is a large double-stranded DNA virus. Following primary infection, usually through mucous membranes of the mouth, it lies dormant in neurones, from where it may be reactivated, often causing 'cold sores' on the lips. The neurotrophic nature of this virus makes it a candidate for gene therapy in neurological disease. HSV-1 vectors can infect non-dividing cells and are not integrated into the host genome.

Adeno-associated viruses

The adeno-associated virus is a small, non-pathogenic parvovirus. It is incapable of autonomous replication, requiring coinfection with another virus (either adenovirus or herpes simplex virus). Because of its small size adenovirus associated vectors can only accommodate DNA inserts of less than 5 kb. Adeno-associated viruses are unique in that they integrate into a specific site on chromosome 19. The discrete integration site reduces the risk of inappropriate gene activation elsewhere in the genome. It infects a wide range of cells, making it a good candidate as a gene delivery system in the CNS.

Lentivirus

Lentiviruses are a subclass of retroviruses that can infect both proliferating and non-proliferating cells and can provide efficient transfer of genes to the CNS. Concerns have been expressed over their safety. These relate particularly to the risk of reversion to wild-type virus, and the potential for mutagenesis at the site of their insertion into the host's DNA, leading to oncogenic transformation.

Non-viral delivery systems

Concern over the safety and potential immunogenicity of viral gene transfer systems has led to the development of non-viral delivery systems. The simplest of these is the administration of naked DNA. Plasmid DNA injected directly into muscle can be taken up and expressed by myocytes, providing a potential mechanism for the treatment of genetic diseases of skeletal muscle. To improve the efficiency of gene transfer, a number of methods for encapsulating plasmid DNA have been developed. Liposomes are synthetic vesicles composed of a lipid bilayer which fuses with cell membranes. Cationic lipids and polymers can also form complexes with DNA in a way which facilitates incorporation into the cell, without the need to encapsulate the DNA. Delivery of DNA into the cell and its transfer to the nucleus can be further enhanced by incorporating viral components which promote cell entry or nuclear targeting. Liposomal-mediated gene transfer has been used in human gene therapy trials of cystic fibrosis (p 104). Although it is less efficient than adenoviral vectors, it appears to lack the toxicity and immunogenicity reported with adenoviral vectors.

Results of clinical trials have so far been a disappointment, with little progress since the first gene therapy clinical trial for adenosine deaminase

(ADA) deficiency (p 101) began in 1990. A major setback occurred in 1999, when an 18-year-old boy died from multiple organ failure four days after starting treatment in a gene therapy trial for ornithine transcarbamylase deficiency, an X-linked disorder of the urea cycle which causes accumulation of ammonia. His death was attributed to an immune response to the adenoviral vector. A further setback occurred with reports that children participating in a gene therapy trial using retroviral vectors in blood stem cells to treat X-linked severe combined immunodeficiency had developed a leukaemia-like illness.

Gene therapy remains experimental. Integrating therapeutic DNA into the genome so that it is expressed for a long duration of time remains a challenge and the potential toxicity of viral vectors remains a major concern. Furthermore, many common diseases, such as hypertension, heart disease and diabetes, are caused by the combined effects of many genes and so would not be amenable to gene therapy as it is currently conceived.

Bioinformatics and use of the internet in genetics

Web-based resources are proving invaluable for both basic and clinical understanding of genetics. For clinicians, there are numerous web sites that provide comprehensive information about clinical features and diagnostic testing for a variety of genetic disorders. Several sites that we recommend include:

http://www.ncbi.nlm.nih.gov/entrez/omim/– Online Mendelian Inheritance in Man (OMIM), includes clinical summaries and details the progress in identifying the molecular basis of disorders; supported by NIH.

http://www.Genetests.org – includes summaries on clinical findings, molecular basis of disorders, as well as links to available diagnostic laboratories and patient/parent support groups; supported by NIH.

http://www.cancer.gov/cancertopics/pdq/genetics/ – detailed summary of genetic aspects of cancers, provided by the National Cancer Institute of NIH.

http://www.kumc.edu/gec/geneinfo.html – provides links to a large number of sites pertaining
to clinical genetics, cytogenetics, genetics edu-
cation and other resources.

http://www.ensembl.org/ – provides free access to
all the data and software from the Ensembl
project, a joint venture between the European
Bioinformatics Institute of the European
Molecular Biology Laboratory and the
Wellcome Trust Sanger Institute. It provides a
powerful analytical browser for the human
genome and other genomes.

http://www.ncbi.nlm.nih.gov/entrez/query.fcgi –
This NIH site is excellent for finding information in the biomedical literature (PubMed),
genomes (human and other, SNPs, STS, etc.),
proteins (sequence and structure), disease
genetics (OMIM) and more.

http://genome.ucsc.edu/ – This site at the University of California at Santa Cruz provides an excellent browser for the human genome sequence.

Impact of molecular biology on genetic diseases

Once a gene has been fully characterized, disease-
causing abnormalities can be identified in both the
DNA sequences and the encoded protein. This
often leads to an improved understanding of the
disease process. Ideally, mutation detection can be
offered as a diagnostic test using DNA samples from
patients who have or are susceptible to the disease,
carriers of the disease and the unborn foetus. Being
able to diagnose a genetic disorder is important for
many reasons such as management of existing
medical problems, prevention of anticipated problems, prognostication, recurrence risk and family
counselling. Specific treatments for many disorders
are not currently available. For these conditions,
accurate genetic diagnosis allows patients to be
educated about the cause of their disorder and provides estimates of the risk of recurrence (genetic
counselling) and genetic testing, when available.

Prenatal diagnosis

Prenatal diagnosis to detect foetal chromosome
abnormalities, genetic mutations and structural
birth defects is widely available. Foetal samples for
chromosome or DNA analysis are generally
obtained by one of three methods:

1 Amniocentesis: This procedure is performed
between 15 and 18 weeks' gestation, and involves
aspiration of amniotic fluid using a needle passed
through the maternal abdominal wall. The fluid
contains cells shed from the developing foetus,
which are used for chromosomal and DNA analysis. In addition the fluid is assayed for components
such as alphafetoprotein, which is elevated in
spina bifida. The risk of procedure-related complications is low, with the most severe complication
of miscarriage occurring ~1/200 cases.

2 Chorionic villus sampling (CVS): This procedure
is done between 10th – 12th weeks of pregnancy
by obtaining a small biopsy of the chorion. The
chorion is a layer of foetal extra-embryonic tissue
that spreads over and invades the uterine wall during early pregnancy. The procedure is most often
performed by inserting a catheter through the
vagina into the cervix of the pregnant uterus. The
miscarriage rate is 1–2%, which is slightly higher
than the rate associated with amniocentesis. An
additional small risk of CVS, if performed before 10
weeks of pregnancy, is limb defects but these
abnormalities do not appear to be increased over
baseline if CVS is done after 10 weeks.

3 Foetal blood sampling (umbilical blood sampling or cordocentesis): In specialized centres
foetal blood sampling is performed under ultrasound guidance to obtain blood from the umbilical vein of the developing foetus. It is associated
with an ~2% risk of miscarriage.

Screening for chromosomal abnormalities, such
as trisomy 21 (Down syndrome), is routinely offered
to 'high risk' mothers due to advanced maternal age
or a previous history of having an infant with a
chromosome abnormality. If the foetus is at
increased risk for having a genetic mutation, analysis is possible if the DNA sequence of the gene of
interest is known and if mutation testing is clinically available. If the exact location and sequence of
the gene are unknown, the probability that the foetus inherited a mutant copy of the gene can be
determined by linkage analysis. This requires DNA
from other affected family members for comparison

of nearby genes or polymorphic microsatellite markers that are closely linked to the gene of interest. Linkage analysis is being used less frequently as the sequences of more genes are identified.

Since the foetal sampling methods discussed are not risk-free, less invasive methods of screening for foetal abnormalities have been developed.

Ultrasound is widely used for assessing foetal growth and development. With the improving resolution of ultrasound, it provides a safe non-invasive method of screening for physical changes such as spina bifida, heart defects, abnormal skeletal development, cleft lip and palate and abnormalities of the renal tract and genitals. Three-dimensional ultrasound and foetal MRI scanning have now been added to the prenatal diagnostic toolbox.

Maternal blood sampling during mid-gestation provides an important method of screening for trisomy 21 as well as structural birth defects. A 'triple screen' uses AFP, unconjugated oestriol and human chorionic gonadotrophin (hCG), in combination with maternal age, weight and gestational age, to estimate the risk of Down syndrome, as well as other conditions. A 'quad' screen, which adds inhibin-A to the 'triple screen' further increases the accuracy of this screening method. First trimester prenatal diagnosis using a combination of maternal serum markers and/or ultrasound landmarks is being developed. The main advantage of these tests is that they pose no risk to the foetus; the main disadvantage is that they are screening tests, not diagnostic tests, and are associated with both false negative and false positive results.

Ethics

The enormous increase in genetics information detailed throughout this book has led to rapid progress in our understanding the causes of single gene disorders and is also beginning to shed light on complex or polygenic disorders. As discussed in Chapter 2, these advances in understanding, as well as in technology, sometimes are double-edged swords raising profound ethical and moral questions (p 85). The guiding tenets of both clinical care and clinical research are Consent, Privacy and Confidentiality. Specifically, a patient's genetic information should be obtained only after receiving explicit consent from the patient and should be considered privileged information that is not divulged to others without express permission to do so from the patient. The US Senate has recently passed the Genetic Information and Non-Discrimination Act that prevents employers and insurance companies from discriminating against persons who have inherited (or are at risk for inheriting) genetic diseases, or who carry susceptibility mutations that increase the risk of developing disorders in the future. Enormous progress in understanding the genetic basis of disease will continue at a rapid pace and these advances hold promise for new treatments. However, concurrent with this progress, we must not lose sight of the individual patient. Accordingly, the medical community must educate itself, as well as engage in development of regulations, to deal with genetic information in a thoughtful sensitive manner that safeguards the individual's right to privacy.

Index

Note: page numbers in *italics* refer to figures, those in **bold** refer to tables.